Gout Relief

Gout Relief and Treatment Through
Natural Remedies

*(Your Quick Guide to Gout Treatment and Home
Remedies)*

Brenda Searcy

Published By **Elena Holly**

Brenda Searcy

Gout Relief: Gout Relief and Treatment Through Natural Remedies (Your Quick Guide to Gout Treatment and Home Remedies)

ISBN   978-1-77485-497-6

Legal & Disclaimer

The information contained in this ebook is not designed to replace or take the place of any form of medicine or professional medical advice. The information in this ebook has been provided for educational & entertainment purposes only.

The information contained in this book has been compiled from sources deemed reliable, and it is accurate to the best of the Author's knowledge; however, the Author cannot guarantee its accuracy and validity and cannot be held liable for any errors or omissions. Changes are periodically made to this book. You must consult your doctor or get professional medical advice before using any of the suggested remedies, techniques, or information in this book.

Upon using the information contained in this book, you agree to hold harmless the Author from and against any damages, costs, and expenses, including any legal fees potentially resulting from the application of any of the information provided by this guide. This disclaimer applies to any damages or injury caused by the use and application, whether directly or indirectly, of any advice or information presented, whether for breach of contract, tort, negligence, personal injury, criminal intent, or under any other cause of action.

You agree to accept all risks of using the information presented inside this book. You need to consult a professional medical practitioner in order to ensure you are both able and healthy enough to participate in this program.

TABLE OF CONTENTS

Introduction

This book outlines proven steps and techniques for treating gout. It includes everything you need be aware of the root causes of gout and determine the most effective treatment for your particular condition.

Gout, an inflammatory joint condition and is a form of arthritis. It's no mysterious illness that only the wealthy suffer from despite the fact that "gout" often brings up images of kings from the past. Gout can be found in around five percent of those suffering from arthritis. It's caused by the accumulation of uric acid within the blood. It is extremely treatable, as you'll read throughout this book.

Whatever your reason the purpose of this book is to provide you with an understanding of the issue and provide solutions to treat gout when it impacts you. The intention and goal in this work is the book can help you, or someone else you love in your life.

1

Chapter 1: What Exactly Is Gout?

Gout can be a painful condition that can occur without warning. For some it can occur following an illness or injury. Gout is identified by intense tenderness, pain, inflammation and redness around joints. Gout is usually felt at the bottom of the big toe, and can spread across other areas. This includes ankles, heels knees, elbows, knees fingers and elbows.

Gout is derived in the French word"gote" and the Latin word gutta which means "a drops". Gout is a condition that occurs when uric acids builds up in bloodstream, and "drops" in joints. This rise in the level of uric acids is known as hyperuricemia.

Uric acid is generally caused by the degrading of purines that can be found in inside the body's tissues as well as in specific food items like beans or liver. Uric acid is usually taken up by bloodstream, moves through the kidneys, and then is removed from the body through urine.

If the level of uric acid is elevated in the body crystals of uric acid that look like needles may develop. If crystals make their way into joints and move, it can be painful, and can lead to swelling. This can lead to gout if it occurs.

The stages of Gout

When someone suffers from Gout, it may be a progression of 4 stages:

Asymptomatic Hyperuricemia - This form of gout is the initial stage. The patient already has an elevated levels of uric acid within their blood. It isn't required to treat or take medication because there aren't any indications.

Acute Gout - In the second stage of gout, elevated levels of uric acids has already caused crystals to build up and become lodged in joints. The person suffering from the condition will notice swelling in joints, which may also trigger extreme pain that is sudden and intense. The attacks that cause pain usually occur during the night, or when one drinks purine-rich drinks or food. In the beginning the acute attack could be present for several weeks and might not happen for a few weeks or even months. However, without treatment, the attacks are more frequent and can become more painful.

Intercritical Gout It is the time between attacks and no symptoms are apparent or felt.

Chronic Tophaceous Gout is a condition that develops over a period of about 10 years it is the most difficult to manage of all. Someone who is afflicted by chronic tophaceous gout suffers from joint damage that is permanent as well as kidney problems. To prevent this type of gout, appropriate treatment is needed.

Do Gout as well as Arthritis the same thing?

Many people mistake gout for arthritis. While both are characterized by severe pain in joints, it's important to understand that they are totally distinct.

Arthritis is an autoimmune chronic disease that is a degenerative disease, whereas Gout is a metabolic disorder.

Gout is defined by pain and swelling of the joints due to crystals of uric acids that build up. Arthritis is caused by joint inflammation. There are various forms of arthritis due to crystals that have formed caused by sodium urate or calcium phosphate. However, they are not urinary.

The joint that is affected by those suffering from Gout usually is swollen, hot, and red. Joints affected by arthritis are also painful and swelling however, they tend to be stiffer.

The signs of Gout

In addition to swelling and redness of joints, gout may be identified by the pain that an sufferer feels. Starting with the toe that is larger, pain is like dipping the joints into extremely cold water. Sharp punctures can be felt. After that, a tearing or stretching sensation may be felt with the increasing pressure. The affected area becomes very sensitive even to most gentle contact. The pain and swelling could be felt throughout the foot, and fever can develop.

A gout attack may last between 3 and 10 days roughly. At this stage, wearing shoes could be unaffordable. If properly treated the attack will end sooner and avoid the likelihood of another attack.

In some instances, people who have chronic grout may also see white or yellowish lumps beneath their skin. They are actually uric acid crystals, also known as "tophi". They are typically located in the toes, fingers and behind the heel, or at the edge of the ear. tophi can be able to penetrate skin creating sores. Tophi can cause serious joint injuries if not treated.

Chapter 2: Contributing Causes Gout

In normal circumstances, the amount of uric acid is released by the body and the amount it flushes out are in balance. However, there are some factors that can cause uric acid levels to rise. This includes:

1.) Age and gender Gout is more prevalent among men and adults more than women.

2.) Genetics - 20 or more those with gout suffer from an ancestral medical history that demonstrates the condition.

3) Weight Obese and overweight people tend to produce higher levels of uric acids because they have more tissue that needs to degrade.

4.) Medical issues related to renal failure , or the kidney's inability of releasing the most waste (including the uric acid) in the blood. People who suffer from kidney stones frequently suffer from gout since the urate crystals also build up inside the urinary tract if the level of uric acid is high.

5) Psoriasis and cancers, as well as other conditions that speed up cell turnover

6.) The blood pressure of high pressure

7) Diabetes

8) Hypothyroidism

9) Alcohol consumption that is excessive - Alcohol, particularly beer, can hinder the elimination of uric acid from the body.

10.) A lack of Vitamin C consumption. Although Vitamin C is essential in the prevention of gout, excessive quantities can also cause increased uric acids levels.

11) Intake of too much fructose Consuming too much soda can increase the risk of developing gout as high as 85%..

12) Diet Consumption of a regular diet high in purine foods like sardines yeast extracts, mussels and herring may cause or aggrave the symptoms of gout. A diet that is low in calories may result in gout.

13) Medicines: Chemotherapy medications diuretics, diuretics and niacin and aspirin may increase the risk of developing Gout.

Gout Diagnosis

If you have symptoms similar or similar to those experienced by gout, you should make appointments with your rheumatologist right away. It's helpful to note the symptoms you've experienced, the time it began, how long it lasted , and how often it happens. A list of your experiences will help make sure that you don't miss anything out during the interview with your doctor. you.

After the initial meeting the rheumatologist is able to conduct two kinds of tests:

Joint fluid tests - this in-depth test involves inserting a needle into the joint that is inflamed to draw a synovial liquid sample. The fluid is later scrutinized under a microscope to detect any evidence of uric acids crystals.

Blood test - A simple blood test is able to determine the amount of uric acids within your blood. However, blood tests aren't intended to be used solely for diagnosing gout since there are some people who have excessive levels of uric acids who don't suffer from gout-related symptoms.

Chapter 3: The Primary Treatment

For Gout

Gout treatment requires medication. These medicines do not just address the current gout attack but also avoid future episodes and minimize complications too.

As with arthritis, gout medicines vary in impact. The doctor may prescribe medications appropriate to the severity of your Gout attack as well as your age and health condition.

Gout Attack Treatments

Non-steroidal anti-inflammatory medicines (NSAIDs) tend to be the highest commonly prescribed medications given to sufferers of gout. It reduces inflammation and pain in joints due to the condition known as gout. The dose of NSAIDs generally begins high, particularly when you suffer from chronic gout. However, once the symptoms have gone away the symptoms are gone, lower doses can be prescribed to stop any future attacks. Examples of NSAIDs include naproxen, ibuprofen as well as indomethacin.

Be aware that a continuous intake of NSAIDs may increase the chance for stomach ulcers and bleeding and pain for some people.

Colchicine is also efficient in relieving symptoms of gout and reducing the symptoms of gout, Colchicine is typically recommended to those who are intolerant or unwilling to use NSAIDs. The pain reliever can cause nausea, vomiting, or diarrhea.

Corticosteroids: Prednisone and different kinds of corticosteroids can be utilized to treat Gout. Most often, they are prescribed in pill form however, there is also the possibility of having the drug delivered directly to the joint for quicker relief. The dose is suitable for the Gout-related condition, long-term corticosteroids use can result in the bone to thin, and a decrease in its capacity to fight infection and slow healing of wounds.

Gout Prevention Medicines

If you're constantly suffering from gout-related attacks, such as more than once a year, or have more severe attacks than normal Your doctor might decide to prescribe medication that decreases the intensity and frequency of attacks.

Probalan (probenecid) helps improve kidney's ability to eliminate greater amounts of uric acids within your body. This lowers the amount of uric acid present in your blood and prevent more crystals from forming inside your joints. Some of the side effects are stomach discomfort, rashes, and in some instances kidney stones.

Xantine Oxidase inhibitors - This kind of medicine, including Uloric, Lopurin and Aloprim helps to stop or reduce the production of uric acids in the body , thus reducing the risk of developing gout. Some side effects include decreased the function of the liver and nausea.

It is crucial to keep in mind that these medicines should only be taken in the aftermath of a gout attack not during. If you take these medications prior to completing treatment for a Gout attack could result in a new, even more severe attack.

Gout Medication Reminders

All medications to treat gout are effective, however they could be dangerous if combined or taken in defiance of your doctor's instructions. If you suffer from other ailments such as high blood pressure, diabetes as well as asthma, liver or kidney issues it is essential to follow the dosage prescribed by your doctor for the medication.

If you're taking medications but still suffer from attacks of gout, it isn't a sign that they're not working. It could be that you are still adapting to the medications that you are taking, so don't quit using them unless your physician recommends it. Consult your physician about your symptoms and experiencing to ensure that your treatment is appropriate for your specific needs.

If you've taken preventive gout medications and are experiencing a gout attacks for the very first time after a period of time, it is best to visit your doctor right away. The doctor might suggest adjustments to the dose and frequency to avoid the possibility of having a gout attack again in the future.

Self-Care Techniques

If you're currently experiencing an attack of gout it can take just a few minutes for the medication to begin working. To ease the pain you feel there are a few self-care strategies you can practice:

The joint affected should be elevated If you are experiencing gout attacks ensure that you raise your feet as frequently as you can. This will reduce the flow in blood flow to your joint, which reduces swelling and reduces the pain.

Do not put any weight onto the joint if you are unable to sit up with your feet in an episode of gout flare-up, attempt to sit down to avoid applying more pressure on the joint.

Don't move the joint. If you are able to immobilize the joint, you'll feel less pain and less swelling. If you're able to then, you might want to make a splint to your joint.

Ice, no heat - For certain individuals, it's an excellent idea to apply an ice cube on a painful or swelling joint. Others prefer for hot soaks to alleviate the pain. Don't be one of the people who do it. While the cold and heat can be soothing to joints, these temperatures will only increase the swelling and pain. Inflammation can be increased by heat and cold could cause crystals of uric form more quickly. Therefore, avoid the ice and stick with moderate - not extreme - temperatures only.

Remove the shoes - When Gout is a problem, take off your shoes to prevent pinching the big toe. If you're at home, you can go without shoes or wear flip-flops. If you are required to wear shoes, choose shoes that allow plenty of room within the toes.

Chapter 4: Remedies At Home To Gout

It is essential in the treatment of the symptoms of gout. However, did you know that there are many natural solutions that can reduce the inflammation and pain of your gout attack too? The home remedies for managing gout are generally safe and all-natural, which means they have a low chance of causing side negative effects. However it is important to be cautious when using these methods. Do not try anything you aren't certain about, and don't ingest anything is a trigger for your allergies. Conduct additional research about any remedy that you can make at home to ensure you know the risks before giving the remedy a go.

Here are some natural remedies to treat gout you should think about:

Organic Apple Cider Vinegar

The product is described as a"miracle in a bottle, natural apple cider vinegar has become an essential in homes due to its capacity to reduce body odor, eliminate sunburn, treat warts and lessen psoriasis-related inflammation, and much more. Gout sufferers such as you must also stock with apple cider vinegar because it is extremely efficient in relieving pains and pains caused by flare-ups of gout. It is anti-inflammatory and is effective in dissolving crystals of uric acid within the body, allowing for better and quicker secretion.

Take 8 cups of water combined with 2 tablespoons of ACV each morning. It is possible to add honey to enhance the flavor. The flavor of ACV might initially be unpleasant but eventually you'll come to appreciate it.

Lime

A fantastic supply of Vitamin C and citric acid Lime is extremely effective in dissolving the uric acid in blood.

Additionally, it helps strengthen tissues and helps heal joints that are painful.

Juice half a lime , then mix it into one glass of water. Consume the drink at least twice per day to see quicker results.

Consuming other varieties of citrus fruits can also help to reduce inflammation and pain in joints.

Charcoal Paste

Small amounts of activated carbon is a common home treatment for Gout. It is due to the fact that charcoal has qualities that can lower levels of uric acid within the body. If you're not interested in using activated charcoal tablets then you could go with a paste. Purchase the tablets from an apothecary or grocery store.

Make the paste by grinding charcoal into a fine powder. Mix it with a tiny quantity of water till a smooth consistency is obtained. Apply the paste directly to the joint affected by gout to relieve.

Baking soda

To reduce the risk of flare-ups with gout, alkalize your body in order to reduce the rate at which uric acid rises. This can be achieved through drinking baking soda-based mixture. Baking soda is an alkaline component that is able to support the body's pH levels to reduce excess uric acid production.

Mix the juice of one lemon, along with 1/2 teaspoon baking soda. Let the mixture to bubble and fizz. After the mixture has settled in 8 ounces, add 8 ounces water and consume it right away. The mixture could cause stomach pain or discomfort.

Although baking soda is considered safe to consume by the USFDA however, it is recommended avoid eating more than 7 quarter teaspoons of baking powder in one day. If you suffer with hypertension, avoid this homemade remedy since it can aggravate your situation.

Epsom Salt

Magnesium is a mineral that is abundant. Epsom salt is another component which is used to treat gout as well as other arthritis-related conditions.

For a full body massage To get rid of all body pain, add two cup of Epsom salt in warm water, then soak into it for at least an hour until the water begins to lose its heat. It is possible to do this at least twice a week.

Safflower

Safflower is often referred to carthamus tinctorius is a plant that's mostly used in traditional medicines. The flower's properties are quite efficient in relieving joint stiffness and pain and inflammation.

Since safflower must be properly prepared to be effective and safe it is recommended to purchase capsules of safflower that are available in health stores or herbal shops in your region. You should take one capsule per day anytime you experience an onset of gout.

Devil's Claw Root

Another well-known herbal medicine is Devil's Claw Root. The name may be scary, but this plant is rich in harpagosides which can improve digestion and ease inflammation and pain that is due to arthritis and gout.

Devil's Claw Root is available in tea, tincture as well as capsules. To help relieve flare-ups from gout the Devil's Claw Root in capsule form is recommended. Each capsule has minimum 50 mg Harpogosides. It is enough for stopping the symptoms of Gout.

Devil's Claw Root is not to be taken if you suffer from gallstones, gastric ulcers or diabetes or expecting.

Mustard Seeds

Apart from adding delicious flavor to food items It is also an effective remedy for gout at home. It is a rich source of magnesium and selenium which reduces inflammation and boosts blood circulation.

Two ways to utilize mustard seeds to relieve gout in two ways - as a paste or as an option for bathing.

The mustard paste is crushed – crush 1 portion of mustard seeds (or you can make mustard powder) and mix it in with 1 part entire wheat flour. Just enough water is needed to make a thick paste. Before using the paste apply petroleum or vegetable shortening jelly to the joint first. Apply a thick layer of mustard seed paste onto gauze and then put it over the joint. Attach the gauze using tape and allow to rest overnight.

Bath soak with mustard seeds - when joints have been affected by Gout it is possible to soak in water containing mustard seeds. Put some mustard seeds on a cheesecloth or muslin and soak in a tub filled warm water. Immerse your entire body or joint that is affected for immediate relief.

Chicory

The spice chicory can be described as both a flavor and a healing herb often present in coffee. It's got many health benefits such as gout flare-up treatment.

You can buy chicory roots at the local grocery store or health store and drink it like tea. All you have to boil is an tablespoon from the plant in one pint water, and then drink it immediately. If you do not like the flavor, allow the drink to cool and then spread it out over the joint, which is painful and swollen.

Apple preserves

Fruity and nutritious, apple preserves help to reduce the accumulation of uric acid crystals within your joints. The preserves, when consumed regularly, can aid in neutralizing the uric acid in your body.

Apple preserves are simple to prepare. After the apples have been cut, peeled and cut all you have to do is simmer in a large pan of water for between 3 and 4 hours. It will be clear that the apples are done when they begin to darken and thicker, as well as more sweet. The apple preserve can be stored in the refrigerator, and eat the same way as jam or other preserve.

Because this home remedy for gout can be sweet and sweet tasting, it may prefer to limit your intake when you have diabetes.

Cherries

It's not obvious but it is a good idea to eat cherries when you're suffering from an attack of gout. The delicious fruit is packed with beneficial properties for healing, including the elimination of toxins and kidney cleaning. Gout sufferers will find that their symptoms diminish faster after eating cherries. Therefore, eat them in whatever shape you prefer whether fresh or baked into the form of a pie.

Blueberries, raspberries, and blackberries are great alternatives if you are unable to locate cherries in your area.

Juniper Oil

Juniper oil is used for many years to offer relief to people suffering from gout, just similar to you. Its healing properties include easing inflammation as well as dissolving uric acid accumulations.

To enjoy the full benefits of juniper oils, all you have to do is rub some drops of the oil into the painful and swollen area for a few minutes. If the joint is painful to touch, soak a small piece of flannel with warm oil of juniper, and apply it to the joint for a couple of minutes.

Ginger Root

Ginger root can be an effective remedy for gout because of its well-known anti-inflammatory properties. There are a variety of ways to use ginger root for gout treatment. You can incorporate it into the various meals you consume, or even eat a tiny portion of ginger root daily. If you enjoy taking tea in the morning, boiling small finger size ginger root in the water in a cup makes the perfect drink.

You can also make a paste for medicinal purposes using a tiny chunk from the root of ginger. Apply the paste directly to the joint and allow it to sit for a couple of minutes.

Bananas

Another fruit that is deliciously effective for treating Gout problems can be found in the fruit called banana. Bananas are a great source of potassium, which helps transform hard uric acid crystals to liquid form. When they become watery, these crystals can be easily flushed of the human body. Bananas are also rich in Vitamin C which can help ease pain and inflammation.

It is a good idea to eat 2-3 bananas or more in the event of an onset of gout to speed up healing.

Chapter 5: The Lifestyle Changes

The use of prescription drugs and home remedies are extremely effective in controlling Gout. To reduce the frequency of flare-ups triggered by gout, and reduce the likelihood of attacks in the future you should make lifestyle adjustments too. These changes in your lifestyle do not just aid in the fight against gout, but also aid in getting healthier throughout your life.

Healthy Weight

The weight of your body increases the pressure on joints and increases the likelihood of having a gout attack in the future. To avoid this, ensure you keep an ideal weight. If you're planning to shed some pounds or drastically reduce your weight, make sure to slow down. Avoid diets that crash and stick to a diet low in purine which is rich in protein, but not high in calories.

Exercise Daily

If you're experiencing discomfort, it's normal to cease activities that appear to stress joints or hurt areas. In the case of gout and arthritis, it's best to exercise until the most severe of the symptoms are over. Moving joints reduces the pain and stiffness, and increases the strength of muscles. The most important thing to do when exercising with gout is sticking to low-intensity activities. Swimming, walking, and biking are the best options for your needs. Begin slowly and keep the workouts shorter. If you do not feel pain but do notice improvements in performance then you could extend your workout, or do more intense workouts.

Increase water intake

Drinking 8-10 glasses of fluid daily keeps your skin healthy , and aids in flushing out uric acid that is accumulating as well. If you consume plenty of water and drink plenty of water, the chance of developing kidney stones will be less likely.

Avoid Alcohol

The research has proven that alcohol triggers the body to store the uric acid, instead of releasing it. If you're looking to prevent any future attacks of gout it is time to stop drinking alcohol and beer. Although alcohol doesn't appear to cause gout however, it is recommended to avoid drinking it as well.

Keep your feet warm

Gout can be a trigger in colder weather, particularly in the event that you allow your feet to freeze. Make sure you wear thick socks and appropriate footwear when it gets cold.

See Your Doctor

Regularly scheduled checkups, even if there isn't an attack in the past, can aid in ensuring that you are on the right path to prevent gout. In these visits your doctor will be able to assess your progress and address any questions. It is also the ideal opportunity to discuss the various options you have to take to reduce the frequency of your gout attacks like using herbal remedies, working out and changing your diet.

Relax

For certain people the stress of life can cause the onset of gout. If you're constantly subjected to stressful situations make time to unwind and relax even for a few minutes each day. Lay down or sit in a comfy position in the most peaceful area of your house. Take a deep breath, relax and let your thoughts go gradually. Keep doing this until you are relaxed. It is possible to also do yoga routines that are simple to master.

Take control of the pain

Gout attacks can cause the pain of a few and discomfort. To get through these episodes, you need to master the art of controlling the discomfort. If you've taken the correct medication, don't fall for the temptation to take more simply as your feet suffering. Try to distract yourself from the pain by engaging in things or sitting in meditation. If none of that works try seeking relief using various solutions at home. If the pain does not disappear after a few days , or when you're suffering from an illness that is feverish, consult your physician immediately.

Chapter 6: Gout Diet

Alongside altering your lifestyle to help treat gout, it is important to look into diet changes as well. The purine-rich foods cause an increase in the level of uric acids in your body, and you should stay clear of these food items at all cost.

What to Avoid

Seafood - Seafoods are especially high in purine , so they're an absolute no-no for you. If you're really having an urge to eat seafood but don't suffer from signs of gout, you can consume a maximum of 6 ounces. Select small portions of shrimp, salmon, lobster, scallops and crab But avoid tuna, anchovies and herring in totality. These types of seafood are laced with high levels of purine, and eating them could cause gout attacks.

Choose Vegetables - Though those suffering from gout are advised to eat more veggies but it is essential to know that not all vegetables are beneficial for joints. Avoid asparagus, beans and peas. Also, avoid lentils or cauliflower, as well as spinach and mushrooms.

Organ Meats Organ meats, such as tongue liver, sweetbreads kidneys, brains, tripe and more are very high in purine. Their purine content is much higher than that present in fish. This should be avoided at all costs.

Red Meat - Both red and white meats have purines, but the amount found within red meats are greater. Limit your consumption to a small amount of beef and pork and limit your consumption to lamb.

Coffee Decaffeinated or caffeinated is diuretic. This means that it slowly reduces the body's water. If you drink many cups of coffee per day, you could be dehydrated and the build-up of uric acid up in joints will occur more quickly. If you are in need of the caffeine boost make sure to limit it to one cup per day.

What to Eat

Make sure you take in plenty of low-fat fruits and yogurts like grapes, carrots sweet potatoes, pineapples along with butternut squash. Since soda, sweet drinks, and excessive coffee are not allowed limit yourself on to milk that is skimmed, juices that are not sweetened and tea.

Gout doesn't mean you aren't able to enjoy food. It's just that you need to be more cautious about the foods you eat and more cautious with your food choices.

It's tempting to indulge in a costly dish of foie gras but are the pain and discomfort caused by an attack of gout really worth the cost? It's not. So, pick your food carefully.

Chapter 7: Uric Acid Relief

Gout is a condition that develops when there is a high concentration of uric acid present in the blood. Uric Acid is usually broken down, then passed through the kidneys before being eliminated through the urine. Different individuals produce different amounts of the uric acid. Some are too high while others aren't excreted by kidneys.

The excess uric acid creates an accumulation and can form sharp crystals in joints and tissues. These crystals resemble needles and are the cause of inflammation and pain that is the cause of gout. While it isn't easy to stop a flare of gout from coming out, you can find relief by using some home solutions. They can decrease the frequency of flares and help ease the symptoms.

Sometimes it's worth repeated. Here are the top four home remedies to relieve uric acids.

Drink plenty of water

When you drink the proper amounts of water you stop the formation of urate crystals. Gout can be found in joints. Studies have shown that staying hydrated can reduce the frequency of gout-related attacks. The recommended amount amounts to 8-12 glasses fluids per day. If you experience flare-ups, it is important to consume more pure, clean water to assist your body rid itself of the uric acids.

AVOID SUPER PURINE FOODS

Purine is a chemical that is found within the body as well as in some food items. About one-third of the crystals the body produces are from food you consume. If you avoid eating foods that is high in purine, you can reduce the frequency and severity of your gout-related attacks. Purine-rich foods include shellfish, fish, along with red meats. Adjust your diet accordingly. Gout is painful and the pain that comes with an attack isn't worth it.

Protect your joints

If you're experiencing a painful flare-up, it's crucial to be extra careful with your joints. Resting regularly and not putting your feet on the ground is recommended by the Arthritis Foundation. It is also possible to raise the joint affected by using pillows.

It is commonplace to utilize a cane in an injury flare-up. It can help keep the pressure off your injured joint.

If the fabric on your toe causes you to feel uncomfortable, cut off the toe area of the socks. It is also recommended to not put your feet beneath your sheets while going to bed.

Be mindful of your weight

The obese tend to be four times more likely develop Gout. In contrast losing weight will help stop the development of crystals of urate. This is one of the reasons that it is important to watch your weight when you suffer from Gout issues. Lower body weight reduces the stress on joints, and could reduce the levels of uric acids.

Chapter 8: What To Relieve Gout Pain Without Medicine

Gout is a form of arthritis that causes painful, stiffness and pain in joints. The precise cause of the condition is unknown however, experts believe it is associated with the presence of high levels of uric acid in blood. The excess of uric acids creates crystals in the joint cartilage as well as the tendons, which causes swelling, redness and joint pain. Gout is a painful disease. How to ease the pain of gout without taking medication is an important topic of concern for many patients.

The first step when you experience gout flares is alleviate the pain and inflammation. The inflammation can be managed with Apple Cider Vinegar. This ingredient is known to have high levels of acidity that ease pain. When coupled together with honey enhances the body's anti-inflammatory reactions, which reduces inflammation. Ginger root is also utilized for the same purpose.

Baking powder is an additional natural remedy for gout. As mentioned above the cause of gout is excess uric acid levels in the blood. Therefore, by reducing the amount of uric acids within the body, the problem is treated. Baking soda is an basic and it reacts with acids via a chemical process which neutralizes acids. Mix the powder in water and drink it three times per daily schedule for two weeks. The juice of a lemon can be combined with baking soda to reduce the acidity.

Epsom salt is a rich concentration of magnesium needed to function properly in the heart as well as blood sugar control. Epsom salt also necessary to regulate blood acidity, as well as to reduce discomfort and inflammation that result from an attack of gout. Soak the affected areas with warm water that is mixed by Epsom salt. It is also possible to enjoy a relaxing bath in warm water that has been mixed in with Epsom salt.

The benefits of water are numerous for the human body, and controlling the gout condition is among them. Water helps prevent the formation of uric acids crystals through helping the body remain well-hydrated. Furthermore, water aids in helping to eliminate excess acids from the body. Drink at 60 fluid ounces water daily during an attack of gout.

Be aware that the importance of healthy eating is not just for the treatment of gout but also to ensure overall health that your body. Take a balanced and balanced meal and include cherries into your diet. Cherries are known for their antioxidants and anthocyanins that are required to ease inflammation.

Other lifestyle choices include regular exercise, limiting the consumption of alcohol, and eliminating food items that raise the level of uric acids within the body like seafood, red meat, and organ meats are crucial.

By following these suggestions regarding how to ease Gout pain with no

41

medication, you may be able to stay clear of the need for medication to treat this problem. Be aware that taking medications could cause other symptoms when the patient is suffering from other conditions like kidney or diabetes. Try these remedies at home to treat gout, and alleviate the discomfort.

Chapter 9: Definition Of Gout

Gout is an inflammation kind of arthritis. It is characterised by extreme swelling, tenderness, and pain of the affected region. It is most often affecting the big toe, which accounts for approximately half of all cases of gout. However it can also affect other body parts like joints and muscles.

The disease of the King

It's caused by excessive uric acid present in blood, which gets stored in joints of our bodies, creating crystals. Uric acid is derived from purine-rich foods like poultry, meat and fish that is fatty. Gout can be traced back to the past, and was often called"the "disease of the monarchs." What's the reason? because during that time there were plenty of foods which only those in the upper echelons of society could afford. Chocolate is one of them but some meats and ale are also eaten mainly at banquets.

The King Henry VIII of England is likely to be the most famous monarch to suffer from Gout. He was frequently depicted on paintings or in photographs as a man holding a piece from meat on one side, and an alcoholic drink in the other. He was also overweight, and prone to being diagnosed with Gout.

The stages of Gout

There are 4 stages in gout that are Asymptomatic, Acute, Chronic and Interval. The initial stage, known as asymptomatic, is distinguished by higher levels of uric acids in the blood, but there are no other symptoms other than swelling or pain within the patient. The acute gout stage defined by intense pain, which is caused by accumulation of uric acid. The pain can last for several days, but then it goes away regardless of treatment. In the interval phase, you are in the time between attacks. At this point, although there is no symptom as in the asymptomatic stage but the uric levels are still high and the odds of an attack in the future are much greater risk. Tophaceous gout that is chronically recurring formed over a prolonged duration of. At this point, tophi could have been present in skin and within soft tissues.

Tophi is an accumulation of uric acids crystals. It is formed on the skin, around joints and on the tip of fingers , referred to as nodes. It is thought to be a sign of gout, which is an advanced stage. While it typically forms around joints, it could appear anywhere on the body. It's often called chalkstones due to of its chalky white appearance.

The Reasons

The main basis of gout and the attack is the increased levels of uric acids in blood. This is referred to as hyperurecemia. Uric acid is an actual waste product of chemical breakdown in our cells, referred to as purine. Purine is a byproduct of food like meat, poultry and fish with fat. That's why a diet with low levels of purine is recommended for those suffering from Gout.

Apart from the food-related causes of gout, there are various other factors that affect the chance of getting Gout. It can be affected through kidney functions, metabolic syndromes and heredity.

Kidney under Excretion

Urate, which is the salts of the uric acid, are eliminated through the kidney. Under the excretion of urate, it causes uric acid to remain in blood, thereby increasing its levels. If this occurs the uric acid appears as tiny needles when examined can be found in joints and causes gout attacks to develop.

Metabolic Syndrome

Obesity, insulin resistance , and hypertension raise the likelihood of developing Gout. It is believed that weight of the body is directly linked to the development of Gout.

Genetics

Rarely, Gout is inherited. There are certain genes that are transferred from the parent to their offspring, as rare genetic disorders that affect kidneys. However, this is just an extremely small percentage of the chance and there is few studies on the development of these diseases. The family lifestyle is known to impact the children of parents who suffer from gout . The lifestyle of a person can be passed down through the generations and, consequently, make the condition indirectly hereditary. The children of parents with gout are already taking preventive actions by being aware of their diet, monitoring their alcohol intake , and taking exercise as a routine.

Triggers

In addition to the reasons mentioned previously, the attack can be triggered by a variety of circumstances. It is caused by the stress of work or in accidents, as well as strenuous work or exercise, and major surgeries. Although there isn't a single research linking these triggers directly with the illness, the attack is caused by one or more of these triggers.

Signs and symptoms

Gout is typically characterized by the occurrence of extreme pain that occurs mostly at night. The painful sensation is usually focused on a particular region, and most of the times in the largest toe, however it could be located in large joints in the body such as knees, ankles elbows, and wrists. The affected area could be red, swelling and tender. Itchy, hot, that appears to be similar to fever, can be the result of the debilitating pain.

Gout's initial sign is apparent by a high concentration of uric acids in blood. The symptoms of gout vary between different stages.

When you are in the beginning stages of gout it can be asymptomatic. This means that there is no obvious physical sign of the disease , other than the presence of high levels of uric acids in blood. The same is true for the intermediate stage that is the one between the attacks of gout.

It is at this stage that the severe pain initially is felt along with the tenderness and swelling of the area affected. In this stage it is possible for the pain to be gone for as long as two days, and no medication is needed and precautions must be taken to prevent an attack in the future.

In the early phase of gout, which develops over a long time period, typically around ten years tophi can be found in patients. They are the nodes of crystals of uric acids. They are usually formed near joints, at the tips of fingers, as well as at the point of the knees and elbows. But, it can also form anywhere such as in the skin or within the ear canals. Additionally, in the advanced stage, pain may be more severe and be more difficult to relieve. In certain cases the pain may be present for up to two weeks.

Diagnosis

Gout is a classic symptom that , in some instances, the diagnostic test is not any longer required to identify the presence of gout in a person. This is typically the situation of Podagra that is associated by pain of the toe's big. In some instances it is recommended to have a test conducted to rule out other conditions because gout could be mistaken with other ailments, for instance when it comes to Rheumatoid arthritis. Also, if there is evidence of tophi within the skin it may be misinterpreted as Basal Cell Cancer.

These are fundamental examinations that are performed for patients who are believed to suffer from Gout.

Recognition of Urate crystals in Synovial Fluid

The synovial fluid can be described as the fluid that is found between joints. It acts as a type of lubricant that is found between the cartilage and bones. The synovial fluid is tested for the presence of urate crystals is the most reliable method for diagnosing Gout. Finding needle-like crystal of urate when viewed under a polarized microscope can be an affirmative test. It is a difficult test that can only be performed by laboratory technicians that are trained specifically to carry out this test.

Blood Testing

Chemistry - For males, above a plasma-urate level of 420 umol/l and for females, over the plasma urate threshold of 360 umol/l is considered a positive outcome, and is an eminent characteristic of gout.

Hematology - An increase the number of white blood cells in absence of signs of illness is an affirmative test, and can be a sign of gout.

Renal Function - extremely low levels of creatinine clearance are related to Gout. In this instance, the kidney might not be able to eliminate the uric acid from the blood, causing an accumulation of uric acids.

Effects

In the paragraphs in the introduction of this guide Gout is a serious condition. In reality, it's extremely serious and its consequences could have a life-changing effect. The discomfort that comes with this condition is well-known that renders the patient inactive for several days, and most times, they miss many hours from working and with their family.

After the first attack, the patient begins to realize that a second attack might occur. This is when the patient becomes aware of his diet and the things he is doing. It is possible that they are restricted from eating food or doing a variety of things. The sudden change in their lifestyle does not just affect his daily routine, but impact his perspective on life.

Changes in mobility

Anyone who has had the experience of experiencing their first gout attack are more aware of numerous things like long walks and climbing. They are worried that they might not be able to accomplish things by themselves if an attack engulfed them. They are worried about the possibility of suffering from an attack when doing activities such as driving. This can affect people in a significant way and a drastic change can be observed by patients.

Dietary changes

Following the initial attack the patient with gout is advised to adhere to the diet of a lower purine intake. To those who have never had a diet prior to, this can be an extremely difficult experience and may take a time to adjust to. In some instances, the radical changes in diet cause an euphoria or state of shock. Physical signs such as hands shaking may be observed. Also , a change in mood is very obvious.

Lifestyle

Gout sufferers could find himself limited in the things he can perform physically as well as what can be eaten and drink, but also discover that he is unable to enjoy his hobbies prior to when it was discovered that he had the condition. For those who love to have a drink and party every at least once a week may find that they are not capable of doing it anymore , or must be able to drink only a small amount or have a few drinks when they are suffering from this condition.

Outlook

Due to gout, people may be inadequate, particularly if they've already been unable to work due to discomfort. Certain people who are highly motivated might be surprised by the condition and could lose faith during the process. The pain can make people more sensitive to feelings and when bodies or joints become damaged due to being affected by tophi they might be embarrassed of their appearance, and might choose to stay at home rather than going out for exercise.

Gout and its association with Rheumatoid Arthritis

Gout is a type of arthritis, it's often misinterpreted as one of its types, such as Rheumatoid Arthritis. They share similar symptoms and signs. Yes, there's that familiar pain, swelling tenderness and redness. However, that's not all. Gout is one of inflammatory forms of arthritis due to high levels of uric acids. While the Rheumatoid Arthritis is an auto immune condition that targets the sufferer's their own muscles and is caused by a mystery. The root cause, treatment and other features are totally distinct between the two.

How do you determine what one you've got?

Here's a chart that compares between them that clearly shows the vast difference between them.

Gout Rheumatoid Arthritis

The signs and symptoms include intense pain, redness, swelling tenderness, the formation of tophi. Intense pain tenderness, swelling, redness

Big Toe affected area Joints, Big Toe, and other body parts Joints other body parts

Causes Accumulation of uric acids in joints and blood Unconfirmed

Type of disease: Metabolic Autoimmune

Diagnosis of Uric acid levels Inflammatory indicators

Gender typically males and females.

Treatment NSAIDs, Colchicine, steroids, Urocosuric NSAIDs, Steroids, DMARDs (Methotrexate)

Gout and its relationship to the other Metabolic Syndrome

Metabolic syndrome is one of the groups of disorders that are an increase in risk factors for heart disease, diabetes , and stroke. The conditions that are associated with it include hypertension and obesity, as well as a elevated blood sugar levels as well as abdominal fat. It also increases cholesterol levels.

The conditions are present in every patient, but the presence of a single condition is a sufficient sign of a condition.

Though it is not directly related metabolic syndrome has never been linked to Gout. If someone suffers from Gout, there's the possibility that he has metabolic syndrome. This is the reason that a person with gout are at risk of developing heart disease, stroke , and diabetes.

Gout is a common cause of the metabolic syndrome could be due to the causes. Gout, as well as the other metabolic syndrome are caused by the food we consume and our lifestyle. Most often, those who are overweight and physically inactive are the ones who suffer from these conditions.

Gout as well as the metabolic syndrome are both related to the kidney's failure and insulin resistance. The decline in kidney function could result in a lack of removal of waste materials from the blood, which can be the cause of some of these disorders and gout.

Treatment

Treatment for gout is different based on the signs and intensity of attacks. In essence, the medications that are readily available at local drugstores are intended to ease and treat the severe pain. If the main symptoms have been addressed with medication, doctors can prescribe it to avoid the possibility of recurring attacks. There are numerous options regarding the types of treatments you could pick from.

Treatment for Gouty Acute Attacks

(NSAIDs) are nonsteroidal anti-inflammatory drugs. (NSAIDs)

These are the most frequently prescribed drugs for people suffering from gout. They are the most effective medication for acute Gout attacks. It can make someone more comfortable within hours of an attack. But, it shouldn't be prescribed to those with gastrointestinal issues.

Colchicine

Colchicine is an alternative medication that can be used in conjunction along with other NSAIDs. It's also a good treatment for acute Gout attacks. It takes longer time to work compared to other NSAIDs. It is believed to be the most effective when used 12 hours following the attack.

Steroid

Corticosteroids, the most common type of steroids, are used to ease severe pain. It is extremely effective and may be acting in a matter of minutes. It can be injected directly into the joint affected or administered intravenously to patients to the hospital.

Preventive Medicines

In the event that patients experience recurring attacks, doctors will prescribe xanthine-oxidase inhibitors. They act as a an inhibitor of the production of uric acid. The majority of the time, the prescription is for allopurinol or febuxostat. However, there are instances where a contraindication to this drug can be observed. When there is the possibility of a contraindication to xanthine inhibitor medications or if the level of uric acid is not excessively high, urocosics medications can be administered.

Natural Treatment for Gout

Cold Compress

If you are experiencing an attack of gout that is acute, and severe pain can be felt the application of a cold compress could assist in relieving the discomfort if it is applied directly to the affected region. You can place an ice pack directly on it, or use a small piece of frozen ice wrapped in the towel.

Increase intake of water

Water can help flush out the excess uric acid from blood. It is recommended to stay hydrated to stop future attacks.

Low-Purine Diet

In the past, uric acid, which cause gout , are a result of the process of breaking down purine, which is a result of the food we consume. This is the primary reason doctors recommend an extreme change in diet for those who are who are diagnosed with Gout. It is recommended to change to a diet that is low in purine. What is a low-purine diet?

It is basically about cutting down on food with a high amount of purine. There are a variety of low-purine diets that are available on the Internet. It is possible to pick the one that is most suitable for your needs. In this article we'll provide an overview of the foods you can eat and what you should stay clear of in a diet low in purines.

What should you beware of?

There are certain foods that are suitable to eat when you're on the low-purine diet. There are certain foods that you could take a tiny amount of, but in a controlled way. But there are certain foods that are strictly prohibited. They are known to cause gout to worsen and could cause irreparable harm to the body. They are well-known and best avoided from your diet, or suffer the pain of. We are all hesitant to suffer. Therefore, here's the list of things to be wary of.

Meat Group

Bacon, veal, liver, venison, processed meat

Seafood Group

- Anchovies, sardines, codfish, mussels, scallops, trout, herring

Sauces

- Gravy

Drinks

- - Beer soft drink (because of the fructose content)

What is safe to take in moderation?

Meat group

- Beef, chicken, or pork

Seafood Group

Crab lobster, oysters, lobster and shrimp

Dairy group

Eggs

Drinks

Liquor or wine coffee

What is there to enjoy?

Dairy group

- Fat-free and low-fat dairy products, including yogurt and cheese

Carbohydrates-rich foods

Rice, noodles pasta , and potatoes

Fruit and Vegetable Group

All of them

Drinks

A lot of fluids, like water, or juice from fruit

Prevention

While there are medications available at the local drug stores for Gout-related attacks, they are just aim to alleviate the severe discomfort and other symptoms of the condition. This does not stop your body from suffering another attack. It is possible to use uric acid blockers to prevent the formation of the uric acid but you already have uric acids in your bloodstream to begin with. It's because we are able to only accomplish a certain amount.

You'll be amazed to find out that the treatment of gout attacks and gout is mostly practical. These are simple things we can do and adhere to to stop the possibility of a painful attack. What do we can do? might be asking. These are all simple things. Here is an overview of the ways we can stop the onset of gout and attack occurring.

Mind your diet

If you're a member of a family with a history of gout, it is possible to start earlier and ensure that your diet is under control. It is possible to eat anything, but certain foods must be consumed in moderate amounts. However in the event that you've been identified as having gout you need to adhere to the strictest diet. Avoid eating foods that are high in purine. Some foods can be consumed in moderation, but items that are listed as blacklisted must not be part of the diet of any kind.

Make sure to drink plenty of water since it can help flush toxic substances from your body. It's not just about flushing out excess uric acid, it also flushes out sugar and cholesterol which can cause metabolic disorders which are the main risk factors of gout.

Lose weight and exercise

It is a good idea to regularly get your body moving. It's not a reason that you don't have the time to exercise. There are many ways you can get your body moving. For instance, you could take the stairs instead of using the elevator, for instance or walk rather than driving the store close to your home. It doesn't have to be an all-out strenuous exercise. It is possible to do whatever is necessary in order to keep the blood moving.

The weight loss will happen gradually. As we've discussed previously the risk of obesity is a cause of gout aswell being a risk factor for metabolic syndrome. The gradual loss of weight can boost your health significantly. But, remember that the process must be gradual or else your body could be in shock when you shed weight quickly.

Need to get a regular exam

Going to the doctor regularly and following the recommendations of your physician can help prevent the development of Gout. A regular blood test can help determine whether the medicines you're using are effective. If you don't have regular health checks, keeping track of your health's progress is not easy and finding out about any issues could be extremely late.

Chapter 10: Five Effective Methods To Identify Gout Signs And Symptoms

According to WebMD the symptoms of gout can differ based on: (1) where in your body you experience manifestations; (2) how the symptoms manifest as well as (3) when symptoms manifest. This chapter will help you'll discover how to recognize symptoms of gout in a reliable manner. This will help you to determine the most effective solution that addresses the root of the problem and free you of the symptoms for good.

Be on the lookout for these 3 Indicators!

Three (3) indisputable signs of gout, regardless of the location the source, when, or how they occur:

1. The sudden manifestation of joint pain, which can vary from moderate to extreme

2. A feeling of discomfort that lasts for days, or even weeks

3. A warm, inflamed and tender joint, with the skin around the area becoming reddish or purplish in hue

How to recognize Gout

1. Take note of the messages your body is giving you during the night. Gout-related symptoms usually occur in the night. So, waking up during the midnight due to discomfort in a particular location in your body usually on your toes,, could be an indication of Gout.

2. Learn to distinguish the Gout symptoms from those related of other health conditions that could be similar, for example those that are:

A) Osteoarthritis - the difference is that the symptoms of this disease appear and gradually develop, while the symptoms of gout appear suddenly. In osteoarthritis, bacteria are typically found in the joint that is affected, but it is rare for gout to occur.

b) Rheumatoid Arthritis - symptoms occur on every side. It typically be affecting multiple (1) joint, unlike Gout, whose symptoms typically manifest in just one joint.

Additionally Rheumatoid Arthritis has its effect on the wrists and hands, whereas Gout can affect the toes as well as feet.

3. Examine your elbows, ears and hands for any nodules. The presence of nodules could indicate the possibility of gout since it often is not accompanied by the typical symptoms.

4. If you are experiencing joint pain that resembles the pain experienced by other ailments, check for any swelling or changes in the color of the joint affected, i.e. the skin appears pink or red. If you experience pain that is sudden and isn't due to injuries, the chances are good that what you're dealing with is gout.

5. The high level of uric acid can trigger the symptoms of gout. Gout is a condition that can be caused by gout. Mayo Clinic lists the following as the causes that can affect

and raise the amount of uric acid within the body:

A) Drinking excessively of alcohol drinks

B) Family history or genetics

C) Genre and Age

D) Health conditions that affect the body like high blood cholesterol, high blood pressure and heart disease

E) Medicines based on drugs that treat

Specific symptoms

Check out the table below for symptoms specific to the condition:

Chronic Gout

Repetitive attacks of joint pain, typically in the big toe area, ankles, feet, and legs

A series of gout attacks may cause deformity in the joint, as also limited movement or slow mobility

Gout on the Feet

The affected foot's skin expands, and it turns reddish and tender to the feel.

Gout on Your Toes

There will be a sudden feeling of discomfort and pain on your toe's big one, which generally occurs during the evening. Most of the time, the pain is acute and will disturb your sleep. Red/purple skin and swelling are common signs of extreme pain.

A Gouty Hand

There is sensitivity in the joint and tenderness in the skin that surrounds the hand affected. If you tighten your fist or inserting your finger into the skin you'll experience moderate to severe discomfort, and sometimes there is a burning sensation that goes along with the discomfort.

Gout or gout-like symptoms in the Finger

There's a problem when flexing your finger. It is often accompanied by pain, stiffness, discomfort and swelling, tenderness of the fingers, skin sensitivity and even burning sensations when you try to move the affected finger.

Elbow Gout

A sign of a problem is extreme pain that appears suddenly within your elbow. The pain will intensify within the next couple of hours or after 12 hours. The skin around the elbow begins to expand and change color to red.

Knee Gout

There will be a throbbing sensation in your knee pain that is sudden and can last for as long as ten days. Your knee is rough and it may feel warm on the touch. In certain situations, you could develop nodules or skin lumps that are referred to as tophi.

No matter where the swelling and pain are in the majority of cases the body temperature will increase, resulting in an increase in fever. In the next section you will find the most effective natural cures to get rid of symptoms associated with gout.

Find the Best Natural Gout Treatments

Medical science and research are still trying to discover an approved cure for the condition known as gout. The reason for this is that the the treatment of gout that is commonly used focuses on relieving the typical symptoms that include: (a) pain and discomfort, (b) inflammation, and (c) swelling in the area of skin.

What are the reasons to stay clear of drug-based medicines

It is normal for people who is suffering from symptoms of gout to look for painkillers, which usually are pharmaceuticals. In the end, doctors prescribe and prescribe these medications and they are guaranteed to never be wrong.

Wrong! The majority of doctors prescribe medicines based on drugs even for the most basic ailment since that's what their education teaches them. It is not to doubt their education, however not all medicines based on drugs are the best for treating ailments. This is particularly applicable when ailments require the use of repeated or prolonged medication, like with chronic illnesses.

Gout-related drugs based on drugs can cause these side negative effects:

* Gastrointestinal problems

* Skin eruptions

* Headaches and sleepiness

* Breathlessness

* Ulcers

* Fluid retention

* The kidney is not functioning properly and/or the liver

* Heart stroke or heart attack

So in the event that your gout does not require urgent medical intervention, you're better off using natural cures.

Herbal Remedies to Treat Gout

It is advisable to continue to consult with your doctor, regardless of whether you decide treatment for gout with natural. A competent physician will be open to exploring every option and will work together with you to discover the best treatment for your particular condition.

Five (5) five (5) of the top remedies to treat symptoms and stop the recurrence and recurrences of your Gout.

Ginger

Ginger has anti-inflammatory properties that are powerful enough to help treat your gout symptoms safely and effectively. A number of studies have established the effectiveness of ginger when treating Gout. Some of the naturally occurring substances in ginger that reduce inflammation and stop it can be: (a) gingerol, and (b) the shogaol.

Ginger can be used to treat the symptoms of gout in various ways, like the following:

* Create your ginger tea.

* If you're able to take it fresh ginger, eat it as it is.

* Make a topical treatment and apply it on the area affected. Here's a quick recipe:

Ingredients

100g of ginger removed and chopped finely

1.5 cups of drinking water

Procedure

Blend or use a processor to mix the ingredients and blend until smooth.

Make sure you only apply a tiny quantity of paste to the area affected, and allow it to sit for about 30 to 45 minutes. Rinse it off. Repeat this every day until symptoms go away.

Boswellia (Indian Frankincense)

The herb is rich in boswellic acids which can regulate the hormones responsible for pain and inflammation. In addition to being one of the most effective herbal remedies for Gout pain, Boswellia enhances blood flow around the regions affected by the condition.

Here are a few ways to reap the benefits of Boswellia for its natural cure for Gout:

* It is possible to put the oil to the skin. Massage the oil gently into the areas

where symptoms are. Keep away from direct sunlight at least for 24 hours following the applying the oil.

* It can be taken as a nutritional supplement. Find a the highest quality anti-inflammatory supplements that list Boswellia as an ingredient.

Celery Seed

Celery seed helps flush of uric acids through the urine, which prevents its accumulation. This can help reduce the risk of developing Gout. Research has also confirmed the effectiveness of celery seeds in relieving joint pain.

This is due to the fact that celery seed is a natural source of that include: sedanolide (anti-inflammation) 3-n-butylpthalide (dissolves the uric acid). For use with celery seeds,

Sip a cup of celery seeds tea. Here's how to make your own tea

Ingredients

The boiling of a cup

A teaspoon of fresh crushed celery seeds

Procedure

The celery seeds should be soaked in the water that is boiling for around 15-25 minutes.

* You may also decide to use it as a supplement to your diet. It's on the market in capsules. Make sure to purchase from genuine sellers.

Devil's Claw

A plant that is abundant in anti-inflammatory properties. devil's paw is renowned because of its ability to get rid of pain that comes with inflammation and gout. It is also an natural cleanser to break down urinary crystals and reduce the build-up of uric acids in the body.

The best method to make use of devil's claw for an natural treatment for gout is to make tea with it. Here's how:

Ingredients

Half one teaspoon of powdered devil's paw root

The boiling of a cup

Procedure

1. Include your claw of devil into the boiling water in the cup.

2. Allow it to steep for 10 to 15 minutes.

3. Take a cup of tea every day until symptoms go away.

Cayenne Pepper

This herb is an effective natural painkiller for Gout. It is an ingredient that is natural and helps in getting rid of inflammation. Indeed, an effective Gout remedy sold in stores uses cayenne pepper as its primary ingredient. You can make your own remedy using natural ingredients by using this recipe

Ingredients

A teaspoon of cayenne pepper

One cup of water

A cup of cider vinegar made from apples

Procedure

1. Bring the water to a boil.

2. Include the vinaigrette.

3. Add cayenne pepper.

4. Cool the mixture before applying it on your Gout.

Natural Home Remedies

Here are a few of the top do-it-yourself home remedies for treating your Gout symptoms:

Epson Salt

The mineral is able to eliminate harmful chemicals from the body. It's a rich source of magnesium, and is essential to maintaining the health and function of your joints and muscles. Based on research from research conducted by the University of Pittsburgh Medical Center the magnesium mineral is active as a muscle relaxant as well as pain relief for gout.

To begin reaping the benefits of Epson salt as a pain relief for Gout, follow these steps:

EPSON SALT WATER FOOT SOAK

1. Then fill up a large and deep tub (or bathe) by filling it with hot water. The amount you fill it with should be enough to fill your feet to the ankles.

2. 0.5 cup of Epson salt added to the water. Let the salt dissolve.

3. Soak your ankles and feet in salted water for about 30 mins to one hour. If the water gets cool then add hot water until you attain the temperature you want or desired warmth.

4. Once the time is up Dry your ankles and feet well.

Lemon Juice

Citric acid from lemons will dissolve uric acid, which causes gout. The process of dissolving uric acids and preventing it from building up in your blood is crucial not only for fighting gout , but also to safeguard the kidneys of your patients. Lemon is a potent neutralizing agent that can help to maintain an optimal acid-alkaline balance.

There are many ways to make use of citrus juice, which is a great natural treatment for Gout. One is to drink lemon-infused water each day upon waking awake in the early morning. Here's a quick recipe:

Anti-Gout Lemon INFUSED Water

Ingredients

1 medium-sized lemon

1 liter/quart of purified water or distillated water

A little grated ginger

Procedure

1. Fill your glass or mason jars with dietary water.

2. Rinse and wash your lemon well. Cut it into thin slices; make certain to get rid of the seeds.

3. Drop the lemon slices into the water. Incorporate your grated ginger.

4. Allow it to sit for at minimum 6 (6) for at least six (6) hours. You may choose to

drink it straight up and add ice or put it in the refrigerator to chill it first.

After drinking your lemon-infused drink, be sure to wash your mouth using clean water, or to clean your teeth. Brushing or rinsing your teeth will stop the acids from lemon from damaging the tooth's enamel. Another method to protect your teeth is using a straw when drinking your lemon-infused drink.

How to treat Gout and achieve the Most Effective Results

Nobody wants to suffer the symptoms of Gout. You wouldn't want that it happened to those who pisses you off. The pain is simply too much.

In the preceding chapter, you learned about how to treat the symptoms associated with gout, without having the use of pharmaceutical medications. This chapter we will focus on the best way to manage gout effectively and avoid it from returning.

What is the cause of Gout?

The most effective method of treating any condition, including gout, is to tackle the root of the issue. What is the reason for Gout? What is the reason you're suffering from its symptoms but others in your family or within your neighbors aren't?

Factors like genetics and alcohol consumption, as well as a bad living habits such as poor eating habits , lack of exercise, stress and other factors can increase the risk of developing Gout. Yet, regardless of the risks, your quantity of uric acids in your body is likely to become the main reason for gout attacks.

If you have high levels urinary acid in your body, which persist for many years, then you could be a prime candidate for flare-ups of gout. This is particularly true when you suffer from hyperuricemia. According to experts from the WebMD as well as the Mayo Clinic, gout results due to "an excess of uric acids within your body".

A surge in uric acid occurs when: (a) your body's systems produce too much the acid and (b) your system fails to flush it out through your urine. What happens is the accumulation transforms into sharp crystals inside your joints, or in the adjacent tissues. This is the reason why you experience pain that is excruciating during an episode of flare-up.

Gout is a condition it's an ongoing condition, just like they are chronic. If you don't treat it in a timely manner at the source the buildup of uric acid will continue until it causes joint disfigurements or even destruction that can lead to damage to both the liver and kidneys.

The Most Effective Treatment

Diet is the most important element that affects the amount of uric acid within your body. What you eat each day could determine the risk of building up uric acids which, could, in turn, cause the development of gout. So, for treatment to be successful you must be able to concentrate on your diet and nutrition in preventing and controlling the development of uric acid crystals.

Find out your nutritional needs

The quality of your food is crucial in fighting off your battles and eventually winning the fight against Gout. The primary cause of the condition is elevated glucose levels in the blood (glucose) which is a typical result of poor diet.

Indeed, a number of studies have confirmed and established the connection between uric acids and glucose, including the study that saw its results publication in May 2012.

Find out what your metabolic or nutritional type is, so you can consume a diet to satisfy your nutritional requirements. It is possible to take the nutritional typing test that is free conducted by the Dr. Joseph Mercola.

Through nutritional typing to nutritional typing, you can determine whether you're:

* Carbohydrate type is that is characterized by high carbs, low protein and a low amount of fat

* Protein type - is defined by high protein levels, fats that are high, and low carbs

* Mixed type is distinguished by a mixture of two types

If you are aware of your nutrition type and type, you can select the appropriate diet to help you fulfill your nutritional needs to the maximum extent possible. When you eat right, you will enjoy good health , including the treatment and prevention of ailments and health conditions Gout is one of them.

Limit the consumption of Alcohol

NHS Recommendation

"Men shouldn't consume greater than three to four units of alcohol per day

Women shouldn't consume more than 2 units in a day

If you've experienced a significant drinking night, stay clear of drinking alcohol for 48 days.

"Regularly" refers to drinking the quantity every day or on most times of week. "

Information Source: NHS Choices

If you enjoy drinking alcohol-based drinks Then this procedure is essential as part of your successful treatment for Gout. There is a lot of evidence that shows that alcohol consumption can increase the risk of suffering from gout because it can increase blood levels for uric acids and insulin. It is therefore recommended to staying clear of drinking alcohol.

Here are some suggestions to help you limit your consumption of alcohol:

Clean your home of alcohol-related beverages. This will reduce the temptation to drink in a comfortable setting in your home.

Increase the strength of your support system. Friends and family members can help you motivate and encourage you to reduce or quit drinking alcohol.

Create small targets and be sure to reward yourself every when you reach your objectives. Small changes can help you to cut down or eliminate your drinking habits.

Get More Physical Activity

As the signs of gout are on their maximum, it can be difficult in moving your body. What can you do to increase the intensity of your exercise help with the gout problem? Moving your body, for instance through exercise improves the flow of blood. This is vital to maintain the proper levels of uric acids. It should be a an integral part of your routine to avoid the recurrence of gout.

So, exercising or increasing physical activity can be beneficial as a preventative measure against attacks with gout. It is recommended to wait until your condition is controlled and your symptoms diminish and fade before beginning exercising to prevent gout.

How to Benefit by Diet for Gout

Your diet could be the best single option to manage the symptoms and stop the recurrence of gout. There is no treatment or cure for gout is ever effective without a nutritional diet as the basis. Therefore, you should begin your treatment by following a gout diet.

What are the reasons to start your Gout Diet

A nutritional deficiency resulting from eating food items that fall under the Standard American Diet (SAD) is the most significant reason you, and many others, suffer from Gout. The processed and junk food is consumed regularly triggers the build-up of uric acid and eventually forms crystals which cause symptoms of gout.

Food that is processed or junk has high levels of purine. In the process of digestion, which is breaking down foodstuffs, the purine transforms into an acid called uric. The excess uric acid alters your blood sugar levels and transforms to "needle-like crystals" that cause lots of problems for your joints. A major cause of this is Gout.

Furthermore processed and junk foods are also high in sugar which includes High fructose Corn Syrup (HFCS). This kind of sugar in food can cause the levels of uric acid to rise and in the event of this, you could most likely expect the symptoms of gout to show up. Unfortunately, the majority of processed foods contain HFCS as it's sweeter than regular sugar, and also costs less.

Dietary advice for Gout

Although there isn't a prescribed or standard diet for gout, you will benefit you to follow an anti-inflammatory eating plan and know which foods to eat and avoid in order to prevent and treat gout. The WebMD experts have a great checklist for this.

In addition to knowing what foods to eat, and what to stay clear of There are other diet changes that could aid:

• Increase your intake of natural and whole foods and limit or reduce your intake of processed food. Avoid junk food.

* Do not drink caffeinated drinks and quit drinking coffee as suggested by Dr. Andrew Weil.

* Increase the amount of fresh, pure water to flush out harmful substances and also to promote the passage of uric acid through your urine.

* Follow your nutritional guidelines. It's beneficial to determine the type of food you consume and plan your eating habits based on it.

Consume fresh juice of pineapple in order to remove your gout-related symptoms. The stem and juice of the pineapple are rich in bromelain, which is a digestive enzyme that helps fight swelling and inflammation. You can also get this enzyme from top quality nutritional supplements.

Reduce the amount of non-vegetable carbs. One option is to replace these carbohydrates with healthy fats including polyunsaturated and monounsaturated fats. Select healthy oils like olive oil and coconut oil that is pure. Olive oil is ideal for dressing salads, and coconut oil that is pure is ideal for cooking.

Additionally to that, you should:

Control your weight. If you've reached the weight you are recommended to maintain, do it by combining the irresistible combination of a healthy diet and consistent exercise. If you're overweight start to shed the excess weight to get to your ideal weight.
Proven Strategies to Gout Relief

Remember Gout can be a long-lasting and progressive illness. Recurrence is normal and each time gout is recurrent, the symptoms increase. In this chapter, you'll learn about a proven method to provide the long-term relief of gout.

Take pleasure in Tart Cherries and Strawberries

Start by establishing a nutritious diet that is suited to your nutritional requirements or needs. Include strawberries and tart cherries, along with fruit juices like strawberry and cherry.

Research has proven that strawberries and cherries can be effective in relieving the symptoms of gout. Their efficacy can be comparable to or exceed the results of aspirin and other pain relievers or anti-inflammatory medications prescribed to treat gout.
What is it that makes strawberries and cherries powerful in their anti-gout remedies?

* The anthocyanin in tart cherries has been proven to be effective in relieving inflammation more effectively than aspirin.

Cherries also contain a significant amounts of bioflavonoids. And together with anthocyanin these antioxidants can help stop and reduce arthritis and gout.

* Strawberries, just like cherries, are high in antioxidants, which protect the body from damage caused by free radicals as

well as the effects of inflammation on tissues of the body.

* The acids found in strawberries dissolve uric acid and also its magnesium content can help the body fight inflammation.

Beware of Stress that isn't needed

Stress can cause your uric acid to increase, and inflammation to become beyond control. Remember that in a certain degree your body requires tension and swelling. It's when they go too much that the problem begins to manifest itself as illnesses and diseases like gout.

Therefore, it is essential to know how you can control stress because it will not only free your body of symptoms associated with gout it will also relieve you from other health issues. It is because doctors across the globe acknowledge that stress is a major contributor in the development of to more than 85% of the diseases.

Improve Your Sleep Habits

Enhancing your sleep habits won't only assist you in managing stress, but enhance the overall health of your body. In reality, quality sleep is non-negotiable in the pursuit of healthy living.

No matter how effective your diet is at controlling gout disease, when you body isn't sleeping enough (quantity and quality together) it will risk exposing yourself to gout , as well as other health issues.

In the sleep phase, the body heals, recovers and restores its best functions. It's like regenerating your health every morning after waking after a great night's sleep.

Start by following this plan to get long-term relief from Gout. Gout relief is achievable by paying attention to the messages your body is giving you. A balanced diet, more physical activity, and enough rest are the only way to help you escape the ravages of gout.

Chapter 11: Understanding Reasons That Cause Gout

Gout typically occurs due to an increased quantity of acid, also known as uric acid in the blood. It can be very difficult and nearly impossible to remove uric acids by excretion if it is accumulated in large amounts. The accumulation of uric acid results in the formation of crystals of urate. This process of crystallization takes place when there is too much Uric acid present. The crystals form within joints of the body, leading to joint swelling and pain, inflammation and soreness. Tendons in joints can be affected due to gout, and cause a decrease in range of motion and flexibility.

Insufficiency of the kidneys, metabolic problems chronic anemia and genetic issues are all risk factors that can contribute to the development of this condition. Obesity is a major risk factor. Because overweight people are afflicted with arthritis, research has shown that obesity could be the cause. People who are overweight tend to produce more uric acids in the bloodstream. Obese patients who suffer by gout are usually injured in joints as a result of crystallization.

As with children and young adults, individuals over 50 years old are more likely to suffer from this condition. It is rare for children to be affected. Incredibly, men suffer from more frequently than women. However women who go through menopausal changes may be affected. Certain people who undergo treatments for a prolonged amount of time with diuretics can be affected by Gout. Patients who have undergone surgery and have suffered from certain illnesses that affect the blood flow are at a higher risk of developing gout. Excessive medical procedures that involve chemotherapy or radiation therapy can be a factor in the risk.

Because gout is a disease that can be passed through generations It can be believed that it could be genetic. Studies have revealed that some people who suffer from gout, also have an ancestry with Gout-related issues.

It is vital to take the appropriate measures to prevent the onset of Gout as there is no specific cure available. To prevent and treat gout, regular exercise and a healthy lifestyle and a balanced diet are vital. While alcohol and smoking consumption are not the cause of gout, they can trigger the symptoms. It is therefore recommended to stay clear of alcohol and tobacco in order to avoid this condition.

Foods that contain high levels of purines and saturated fats could affect the amount of the release of uric acids. Purine is synthesized by our bodies, then uric acids is released in larger quantities to the bloodstream. Therefore, it is recommended to avoid eating foods like fish and organ meats that have purine. Certain dairy products and even vegetables also contain large amounts of purine.

The most suitable foods for those who suffer from gout include cereals, chicken and milk that are low in fat fruits, as well as the green vegetables. It is easy to eliminate uric acid through drinking plenty of water. Aiming to drink two liters of fluid daily is suggested to assist the body eliminate the uric acid effectively.

Gout sufferers may suffer from abrupt and sudden pain that can recur frequently. These episodes could be the first indication for chronic gout. Certain people suffer from extreme pain during the night, and not during the daytime. There is a variant of gout called pseudo gout. This is typically caused by crystallized calcium being deposited in place of the uric crystals within the joints.

Understanding Gout Attacks

Gout typically affects older and middle-aged people, and rarely affects younger individuals. While gout-related conditions can be found for both genders, the prevalence is more prevalent for males. It has been found that women suffer from this condition more often following menopausal changes.

Gout is caused by the crystallization of uric acid to form sharp, jagged structures in blood. These tiny crystals are the major cause of the severe swelling coupled with pain that gout has become well-known for. This is why it is crucial to know the causes for uric acids formation and the accumulation of bloodstream and recognize the symptoms of gout in the event of.

Gout-related symptoms are similar to those that are seen in rheumatoid arthritis. The majority of sufferers experience extreme discomfort in their surrounding connective tissues and joints with swelling and inflammation in the lower the limbs. Gout can recur at times and can be chronic in nature. The severe joint pain that is that results from a gout attack can be a short period of hours up to number of days. As the condition progresses and the time frame can stretch by 8-10 days certain instances.

In the beginning, gout attacks typically occur in lower body parts including in the area of ankles, heels and toes. A majority of people who suffer from gout have intense attacks that occur around the big toe. These are referred to as podagra. They typically cause burning, swelling sensations, pain and inflammation. Gout attacks that are severe do not last long, but they are extremely intense in the nature. They typically occur at night and typically last for 3-4 hours. The cause of Podagra is extreme physical exertion or injuries that affect the lower limbs of your.

Gout attacks that are severe are more intenseand last for a longer time and can occur in various parts of the body. Apart from the toe, other parts that are afflicted by these repeated attacks may also experience swelling and pain in fingers, knees, elbows and wrists. Both kinds of gout attacks are likely to cause the sensation of a mild or low amount of sweat and high fever.

The frequency and intensity of a gout attack is affected by many elements like alcohol consumption as well as physical activity, unhealthy diet, and overweight. To prevent the recurrence of Gout-related pain, patients are frequently advised to limit eating animal flesh and seafood within their specific diet. Additionally, a higher intake of alcohol, especially beer, may contribute to gout because of its an extremely high amount of purine. Raw vegetables dairy items "low in fat" and fresh raw fruits can help prevent the appearance of various symptoms, and can also help in the overall improvement of Gout-related attacks. In addition, those suffering from gout should also be advised to divide their meals into smaller portions and refrain from eating anything before bedtime.

In order to ease the pain of Gout, doctors typically prescribe various anti-inflammatory medications. Patients who suffer from frequent and severe attacks due to gout are advised to receive corticosteroids as an injection because they offer quick relief for joint pain and tenderness. Other medications that aid in preventing repetition of attacks in the future related to gout include sulfinpyrazone and allopurinol. probenecid.

Diagnosis and pathogenesis of Gout

Gout, in the majority of cases, is caused by high level of uric acids in the blood. Uric acid is one of the byproducts from the metabolism process of purine-related components. It is eliminated from the body through kidneys through urine. The presence of excess uric acid in the blood system of the body could be due to issues with the elimination of wastes that make it difficult for the body to rid itself of uric acid. But, the majority of cases of gout have evidence of renal diseases that lead to an inefficient elimination associated with the uric acid.

The elevated levels of uric acids in the bloodstream (hyperuricemia) throughout the body is associated with the presence of gout however, it has not always been the primary cause. There are occasions when people with gout have an acceptable amount of serum uric acids. In addition there are those with a condition called hyperuricemia, but do not develop Gout. Rheumatoid arthritis has a strong similarity to the symptoms of Gout, however, medically speaking, the two conditions do not have any connection.

Gout can be recognized by its symptoms and signs. However, additional medical examinations like blood tests or tissue samples are necessary to establish the condition. To determine if gout is a problem, specific evidence of an accumulation of uric acid on joints and body tissues must be established. A large percentage of patients with gout have the level of uric acid in their blood that is 7 mg per dL or more. It is now known that Hyperuricemia isn't the main reason for gout although the majority of gout patients have higher levels of uric acids within their blood.

A lot of people suffering from gout experience an increase in the uric acid resulting from of consuming foods high in purine. But, the overproduction may be related to other physiological abnormalities. Modern studies have identified several physical abnormalities that could cause Gout. The research revealed abnormal enzyme activity that affects the correct regulation in the production of purine. Gout is also acknowledged as a condition that can be found in bloodlines of patients who have a history of family members of gout.

There are instances where gout occurs due to irregular excretion that has to do with the uric acid. Uric acid is eliminated through the kidneys, or the gastrointestinal tract by the feces and urine. If the kidneys aren't functioning in a way that is appropriate, the proper elimination of waste cannot occur. In this instance, gout could be the result of an illness or kidney disorder.

Gout symptoms that are intermittent include extreme discomfort in joints. The pain can intensify and become worse at late at night, which can last for several hours or days. The medical gout treatment targets two factors: the excessive serum uric acids and painful attacks of gout. The treatment aims to control the control of serum uric acids. When healing is in progress doctors usually prescribe anti-inflammatory (non-steroidal) medication such as colchinide medications, or cortocisteriods injections. Additionally the proper planning of meals and lifestyle modifications will be recommended and advised. As the research on gout in the clinic and medically augmented methods, strategies will be developed likely to be in place soon to overcome the disease and prevent its recurrence.

Gout Treatment and Gout Issues

There are a variety of causes that could trigger the development of Gout. The medical condition develops when your body produces excessive Uric acid. Acid such as this is an insoluble substance that is excreted by the body of a person via urine. The excess uric acid typically builds up and is stored as crystals of uric. The body deposits crystals of urate into joints in the human body. They cause painful inflammation in a lot of gout sufferers and are usually felt in the toes.

It is impossible to treat this condition however there are a variety of effective treatments for gout that can be utilized to ease the symptoms. There are prescription drugs which can help reduce the symptoms of pain, but they are not able to treat the root cause. Changes in lifestyle may be necessary to get rid of the root causes of Gout. Also eating a healthy and balanced diet, quitting smoking and abstaining from drinking alcohol are just a few of the changes people suffering from gout must take. Bad habits like drinking in excess alcohol are known to cause an increase in gout.

A lot of gout sufferers experience extreme joint pain. Gout attacks are typically extremely painful in the late at night and can hinder patients from sleeping. Gout medication prescribed by a doctor doesn't prevent the painful episodes from happening again however, they can be extremely helpful in the short-term reduction of these episodes.

The most popular types of drugs prescribed to treat gout comprise anti-inflammatory (non-steroidal) medications, which are also known as NSAIDS. The names that are generic include ibuprofen, indomethacin, diclofenac ketoprofen and naproxen. These medicines work well in reducing swelling associated with pain that is associated with the illness. Anti-inflammatory medicines are generally accepted by the majority of people. They're administered orally, and the dosages are generally recommended by a doctor.

Another medicine that could be utilized to fight the gout condition is Colchicine. This medication reduces pain significantly in areas of the body affected by gout, however there are some negative side consequences. This is why Colchicine is generally prescribed to patients suffering from severe gout, or who is unable to take anti-inflammatory (non-steroidal) medication.

Corticosteroids may also be used in the treatment of Gout. This form of treatment offers quick pain relief, and is injected directly into the joint affected by the injury. Since corticosteroids can cause negative adverse side negative effects, these injections should be reserved for those with severe gout-related conditions.

Consuming a lot of quality water and following an appropriate diet are both natural methods to rid the body of unwelcome uric acid. Certain medications can be prescribed to regulate an increase in uric acid levels within the body. These medications are commonly used to treat chronic symptoms of Gout. Allopurinol is an inhibitor that reduces the quantity of uric acids in the body. Uricosuric drugs like sulfinpyrazone as well as probenecid are used to enhance the kidney's function and help them get rid of the excess uric acids.

A lot of people can lessen the pain of gout by taking a gout treatment that is effective. It is essential to be aware that persistent variations of gout symptoms could reappear with time, and this means the treatment for gout may need to be reintroduced.

The relationship to Diets and Gout

Gout is certainly an important genetic component. those who eat unhealthy meals are at a higher risk of getting the disease.

There have been numerous attempts by researchers over the years to prove the connection between diet and the progression and development of Gout. Based on the numerous studies and information collected it is now clear that people who have diets that are largely comprised of fish and other fatty foods are more likely to develop gout. It is confirmed that seafood and meats with high fat content increase the amount of uric acid present in the bloodstream and can trigger the development of gout. However, research has proven that a diet that is unhealthy isn't the only reason for gout, since there are plenty of people who have a poor diet and have large amounts of uric acids within their bodies however, they do not suffer from gout. Therefore, it is possible to say that the progression and development of gout is greatly dependent on other factors, such as the genetics, alcohol intake as well as a lifestyle of sedentary and weight.

Recent studies and studies that show low-fat dairy products can be a major factor in combating and managing the symptoms of gout. According to research, the proteins in milk aid in the elimination of excess uric acid out of the body, which is the main chemical that causes the development and growth of the condition known as gout. There are studies which have revealed that those who consume dairy products that are low in fat are twice as likely to suffer from this condition as compared to those who don't consume dairy products all the time. The experts at nutrition recommend drinking 2 glasses of milk skim every day to help prevent the development of Gout.

Anyone who is susceptible to developing gout should reduce their consumption of fattier meats like lamb, beef, pork and duck. Seafoods are also known to contain a high amount of purine. It is also recommended to be restricted in your diet. Meats that contain organs like kidneys, livers and heart meats should be avoided if at all possible as they can significantly increase the likelihood of developing Gout. In addition, people at risk should be cautious about drinking alcohol as it has been proven to be a factor in the development of gout.

Vegetables are certainly a healthier alternative to meat since they are rich in unsaturated fats as well as high in fiber. But, they could increase the risk of developing gout due to their high content of purines that contribute to the production of uric acid within the body. However eating a balanced diet of fresh fruits and vegetables is much more healthy than one that includes many meat-based products. People who are at risk of developing this disease should consume at least 2 plus liters pure water each day, the recommended daily water intake for everyone, in order to assist in the elimination of excess Uric acid levels out of the body.

The importance of Gout Diets

The Gout diet is a diet program that is offered to patients to lessen the severity of gout-related attacks. The principal reason to follow the strict diet of sufferers of gout is to lower the intake of purine as well as reduce the uric acid levels in the body. Certain types of organisms are required in order to eliminate uric acid out of the body. To do this, gout sufferers should be able to drink around two liters each day, with distilled water preferred and non-alcoholic beverages.

Gout sufferers will probably have uric crystals forming within their urinary system. It's best to get rid of it. If not, it could result in inflammation of your urinary tract. To avoid the overproduction of uric acid patients must refrain from eating kidneys, livers and various organ meats. Consumption of seafood should be cut down in addition to these meals as they increase the body's uric acid production. Also, the consumption of sweets must be cut down. Consider replacing these meals with choosing healthier alternatives like boiling or steamed white meatthat is and not frittered. Steaming and boiling food is superior to frying since it keeps the nutrients in the food. Additionally, the food tastes more sour and not as oily. People with gout can't take in fried food.

The gout diet is effective in treating the disease since it is made up mostly of leafy, green fruits, vegetables, and plenty of liquids. Skim milk, yogurt and dairy products with low fat could also be part of the gout diet because they may help normalize level of serum uric acids and are highly recommended by medical professionals. If feasible, the water to drink by the sufferer should be pure. It is also suggested to drink alkaline water for treating this condition. Alkaline water is processed water that is used to boost the alkalinity in the liquid. It's very efficient to neutralize the effect of the urinary acid within the body.

Complete List of Foods Rich in Purine

Below is an easy reference list of purine-rich foods. Beginning with food items that contain the highest levels of Purine approximately. 400 mg. Uric acid/100 grams or greater. This list can give you an idea of the food items you should stay clear of if you're suffering from gout-related issues.

Foods rich in Purines:

* Sardines, fish, and fish in oil

* Liver, Calf's

* Mushroom flat edible Boletus dried

* Neck sweet bread, Calf's

* Ox liver, spleen

* Pig's heart, liver, lungs, spleen

* Sheep's spleen

* Sprat, smoked

* Theobromine

* Yeast, Baker's, Brewer's

Foods that contain moderate amounts of Purine:

* Bacon

* Bean, seed, white, dry, Soya,

* Beefand chuck fillet, fore-rib Entrecote meat only sirloin and shoulder

* Black gram (mungo bean), seed, dry

* Caviar (real)

*Chicken (breast without skin), (chicken for roasting) "average" cooking fowl "average" Leg with skin, but no bone Liver

* Duck, average

*Fish, Anchovy, Bluefish, Carp, Cod, Haddock, Halibut, Herring (roe, Atlantic, Matje cured), Mackerel, Pike-perch, Redfish (ocean perch), Saithe (coalfish), Salmon, Sardine (pilchard), Sole, Trout, Tuna (Tuna in water, oil and water, etc.)

* Goose

* Grape, dried, raisin, sultana

* Grouse

* Ham Cooked

* Heart, Sheep's

* Horse meat

* Kidney, Calf's

* Lamb (muscles only)

* Lentil, seed, dry

* Linseed

* Lobster

* Lungs, Calf's

* Mussel

* Mutton

* Ox heart, kidney, lungs (lights), tongue

* Partridge

* Chick, peas (garbanzo) seeds Dry

* Pheasant

* The tongue, kidneys of a pig

* Pike

*Poppy seed seed dry

* Pork belly, raw dried and smoked

• Pork chops with bones fillet, chuck, hip as well as the leg bone (hind leg),

Only Pork Muscles

• Pork shoulder skin (blade of the shoulder)

* Meat of Rabbit/Hare, with an average bone

* Sausage "Jagdwurst" Salami, (German) liver (liverwurst) and frying (from pork)

* Scallop

* Shrimp, brown

* Spleen, Calf's

* Spinach

* Sunflower seeds dry

* Turkey Young animal average with skin

* Cutlet, veal chop with bone, fillet Knuckle with bone, leg of veal containing bone just muscles, neck of veal with bones, shoulder

* Venison back, haunch (leg)

Foods with a low amount of Purine:

* Almond sweet

* Apple

* Apricot

* Artichoke

* Asparagus

* Aubergine (Eggplant)

* Avocado

* Bamboo Shoots

* Banana

* Barley with no husk, whole grain

* Bean sprouts Soya

* Beans French (string beans the haricot) , dried

* Beef (German), corned (German)

* Beer, alcohol free, Pilsner lager beer, regular beer, German, real, light

* Beet root

* Bilberry, blueberry, huckleberry

* Brain, Calf's

* Bread wheat (flour) or (white bread)

* Broccoli

* Brussel sprouts

* Cabbage and red white, savoy

* Carrot

* Cauliflower

* Caviar substitute

* Celeriac

* Cheese Brie, Cheddar/Cheshire cheese 50% fat content, Cottage, edam, 30 percent, 40% and 45percent fat content in Dry matter. Limburger 20 percent weight of dry matter as fat

* Cherries, Morello, sweet

* Chicory

* Chinese leaves

* Chives

* Cocoa powder

* Corn sweet

* Crayfish (Lobster)

* Cress

* Crispbread

* Cucumber

* Red currant * Red

* Date dried

* Elderberry, black

* Endive

* Fennel leaves

* Fig (dried)

* Fish, eel (smoked)

* Frankfurter sausages

* Gooseberry

* Grape

* Grass, Viper's (black salsify)

* Kale

* Kiwi fruit (Chinese gooseberry, strawberry peach)

* Kohlrabi

* Leek

* Lettuce

* Lettuce, Lamb's

* Luncheon, Meat

* Melon, Cantelope

* Millet, shucked corn

* Morel

* Mushroom, flat edible Boletus cans solid and liquid Chanterelles cans, solids and liquids

* Nuts, Brazil, hazelnut (cobnut), peanut

* Oats, with no husk whole grain

* Green, olive, marinated

* Onion

* Orange

Ox brain

* Oyster

* Oyster * Mushroom

* Parsley Leaf

* Pasta that is made from egg (noodles, macaroni, and spaghetti)

* Peaand pod, and seed green dry

* Peach

* Pear

* Peppers and green

* Brain of a pig

* Pineapple

* Plaice

* Plum

* Plum dried

* Potato

* Potato cooked with skin

* Pudding * Pudding, black

* Pumpkin

* Quince

* Radish

* Radishes

* Raspberry

* Rhubarb

* Bread, rolls

* Rye Whole grain

* Sauerkraut, drip-dripped off

* Sausage "Bierschincken", "Fleischwurst", "Mortadella", "Munich Weisswurst",

Vienna, frying, from veal, German (Mettwurst)

* Sesame (gingelly) seeds, Oriental, dry

* Spinach

* Squash, summer

* Strawberry

* Tench

* Tomato

* Walnut

* Whole grain wheat, Wheat

* Yogurt, min. 3.5 percent fat content

Proper Gout Diets Prevents and reduces the symptoms of Gout.

Gout symptoms are easily cured and avoided by following a healthy diet that is gout-friendly and having a healthy life style. There is no definitive treatment for gout and the treatment recommended helps ease the pain and inflammation that are caused by the condition. As those suffering from gout realize, there's no medication that can combat the condition, particularly when it is more severe cases of gout. The most effective method of controlling your diet would be to stick to an appropriate gout-specific diet. the proper gout-friendly diet can alleviate signs of gout as as decrease the risk of injuries and complications.

A healthy diet for gout works by eliminating foods that cause gout out of the diet. Gout is caused by food items that have high levels of saturated fats and purines. These foods are substituted with healthier foods that are more easily tolerated.

The high levels of purine are extremely difficult to avoid since they are present in a variety of food items. This includes: pork, beef, lamb chicken, organ meats, poultry, seafood, fish and dairy products that are fatty (cheese butter, butter and milk, etc.). A healthy gout diet has to be planned with care and thoroughly researched. It is possible to think that you're healthy, but you're still eating a diet high in purine. For instance there are many vegetables that contain a high amount of purine including peas, spinach and beans. Even though these foods contain huge amounts of purinein them, these vegetables aren't believed to have any adverse impacts on the body. A diet high in fruits is vital to prevent gout and it is recommended to include fruits in any diet plan for gout. They are the best food as they contain lower levels of purines and vitamins and. For instance Vitamin C acts as an antioxidant which aids in reducing the effect of gout.

While diets for gout do not include a lot of meat however, there are some which can be consumed. This includes chicken and lower fat meats.

A healthy diet for gout must comprise fruits, vegetables and soy as a substitute for cereals, dairy products brown rice, cereals, and bread. It is important to drink enough alkaline water in order to help the kidneys get rid of excess urinary acid.

Dietary Effects and Lifestyles with Gout

If you suffer from gout, they must make some adjustments to the way they eat and live. If, for instance, you suffer from gout and are overweight, it is important to consult with your doctor about a suitable exercise program to reach your ideal weight. Apart from the truth that having a weight problem isn't healthy in all cases, excess weight can cause stress on joints, and can also increase the amount of the amount of uric acids and trigger flare-ups of gout.

Gout sufferers typically don't have the ability to process uric acids so they must avoid any activity that can cause an increase in it within the body. But, do not go into extremes in order to lose weight or start eating a fast. These can result in more uric acids and cause gout flare-ups.

There are ways to modify your diet in a way that will lessen the severity of gout flare-ups by adding the glass of cherry juice or any other purple fruit into your daily diet. Cherries contain antioxidants and help reduce inflammation, which can help stop flare-ups. Also, you can add food items which are rich in Omega 3's such as walnuts, flax seeds as well as the fish oil capsules. Another great thing to eat is low fat milk.

Get plenty of water. This can help rid of the excess uric acids in your body. It is also recommended to avoid alcohol as much as you can because it increases the amount of uric acids in blood.

The main point is that if Gout, you should consult your physician about some of the food restrictions. He will help you determine a suitable diet and also inform you more about these and other food items which can harm and aid in the treatment of the gout. This is especially important when you're one of the people who cannot endure the medicines prescribed for gout and must be able to control it completely through diet and diet alone.

A Gout Diet is low in Purines

If you are eating your diet high in protein and purine high foods, it could result in flare-ups of gout symptoms. So, these types of foods are to be avoided as they could cause uric acid levels to increase. Certain kinds of meats contain purine and therefore should be avoided or consumed in small amounts to reduce the risk of suffering from gout.

Organ meats such as kidneys, livers or brain are purine-rich and should not be consumed. Other food items to stay clear of include mackerel, anchovies, herring and mussels, sardines, yeast, smelt, dried peas and beans. These are just a brief list of foods that are problematic that are available, and more varieties of fish and meats are included on the list of items to stay clear of. If you do decide to eat these types of foods, take more veggies, and most importantly, those who suffer from gout should avoid any protein supplement of any kind.

Gout reports are always negative, and they tell you what to avoid eating in order to trigger an flare-up. But what are some foods to eat that actually aid in avoiding flare-ups? It is said that the American Medical Association has put out a list with the foods they recommend gout sufferers consume. In addition, some of the suggestions include:

Consuming complex carbohydrates, such as fiber-rich whole grains, fruits and even vegetables. Eat around fifteen percent as protein, and less than 30% of your daily calories should come from fats. The fruits like cherries like we mentioned earlier along with blueberries and strawberries are great options to consume if you suffer from gout. It is also possible to eat other foods such as pineapple, bananas, celery, tomatoes, kale , and other leafy vegetables as well as food items that are high in Vitamin C.

Additionally, it's fine to sip tea or coffee and tea, but remember to drinking eight or more glasses of water that is pure in addition.

General Instructions for Gout

If someone has Gout, they naturally need to know what to do about it. Gout is a painful condition that is caused by crystals of uric acid develop in joints. After which, the patient develops an inflammation, and the area starts to swell up, it feels stiff and triggers extreme discomfort. Although everyone is affected by uric acid however, most of us's kidneys can eliminate excess waste urine. But, for those with gout, this process isn't performed in a proper manner.

One of the most common things performed when a doctor has confirmed that someone suffers from gout is treating the pain that is severe with anti-inflammatory pain medicines. The doctor will also prescribe medication to decrease the production of Uric acid. But, there are some who cannot take these medicines, and consequently, they tackle their issues in a more holistic manner by taking steps to decrease the amount of excessive uric acids within their bodies.

This is accomplished by avoiding purine-rich foods since purine is a component of uric acid within the blood. Additionally, they take steps to manage their weight and the overall general health through a healthier way of life and avoiding certain kinds of foods or drinks like the ones mentioned in the previous section about the right diet for people suffering from gout.

Superfoods, Water and Treatment for Gout Relief

Apples are high in vitamin C and pectin which helps to ease the symptoms of gout. Vitamin C boosts your immune system more robust and pectin makes joints flexible.

Onions are potent antibiotics that can aid in the blood circulation. They possess diuretic properties that aid in the treatment of kidney infections and decrease arthritis and rheumatism.

Beets are more iron-rich than spinach, however either of them is beneficial for the body since they function as an organ for kidney filtration and prevent kidney stones from developing. Avoid eating foods high in purine as they are responsible for half your uric acids. It is also recommended to avoid sweet breads, organ meats such as liver mackerel and herring, wild game meat, cauliflower in addition to meat extracts and sardines.

Consuming berries and fruits like blackberries, cherries and strawberries, which are dark colors are identified to aid in lowering levels of uric acid. Because they contain antioxidants and chemical compounds which aid in the reduction of uric acid.

Drinking Water for Gout

One of the best natural cures for this disease is to drink plenty of water. Gout pain can be caused due to crystals that have accumulated within the body. Crystals are deposited and transported into joints, resulting in pain and discomfort. When you drink lots of quality drinking water, it might need to use the bathroom often, however it can aid in eliminating the excess crystals that accumulate in the body.

There are many advantages of H2O for the treatment of gout pain:

1. It helps in the elimination of crystals, as well as other waste.

2. Helps to maintain general hydration.

3. Helps alleviate pain caused by kidney stones.

4. Helps to improve metabolism that aids in losing weight (excess fat may be a factor in relation to pain from gout).

5. Helps to stop more painful episodes of gout.

Gout is actually a result of four phases. The four phases that are that are associated with gout pain tend to be asymptomatic, intense persistent, intercritical, and persistent.

The initial phase that is of gout pain might be the most severe phase. It is usually accompanied by no indications or symptoms This particular phase with gout pain signifies the beginning of crystals that are responsible for the irritation and discomfort that are associated with more advanced phases of the condition.

The initial episode that is associated with Gout pain happens in the extreme stage of this condition. The second stage that is characterized by gout pain can cause moderate and even severe round pain due to gout. Gout pain episodes can last longer than a couple of days.

The first gout pain attack is usually in a period of time that can last for many months, or even years after the condition actually started. This particular phase is known as the intercritical stage and is connected with pain from gout. The majority of people suffering from gout have their second episode within two years after the first time they experience.

If you don't consume enough fluids and your body is dehydrated. In addition, dehydration can trigger other problems such as kidney problems. If the kidneys aren't working properly it can trigger the formation in kidney stones, infections and the formation of crystal accumulation. As you've heard, additional crystals can be the main reason for pain in gout.

It's not just a matter of not drinking enough water. The body could not be adequately hydrated if you drink drinks like teas, coffee, alcohol-based drinks, or even carbonated drinks regularly. So, when it comes to the prevention of gout pain and treatments the first thing you must take is to reduce intake of these kinds of beverages and to improve your drinking water intake.

It is sometimes difficult to drink a lot of water each day. In these cases you can eat fresh fruits or vegetables or fruit juice. But, it is recommended to drink plenty of water at all times to keep hydrated.

Other natural remedies for gout pain concentrate on the foods you like to consume. Are your diet plans a healthy one? You should avoid eating foods that contain greater Purine levels as they could cause the accumulation of crystals.

Other Treatments

One remedy that has been utilized to treat Gout since the 1800's was Colchine. While this remedy can produce positive results, it's not without risks, which include nausea and diarrhea.

Another non-steroidal anti-inflammatory medicine often prescribed to patients suffering from gout is called Inodmethacin. This NSAID is not a part of the same ramifications as Colchine. People suffering from gout should stay clear of using aspirin if they are suffering from an attack.

Patients who experience multiple kidney stones or gout attacks should get their uric acids levels stabilized. One drug that assists in regulating the levels of uric acid inside the kidneys is Probeniced. Alopirnol was developed to block the build-up of uric acid in the body.

A potent medication that is prescribed to patients those suffering from kidney problems as well as kidney stones are Zyloprim. Zylorpim lowers the amount of uric acid produced. However, some patients suffered from side effects, such as an itch on the skin and an stomach upset. The effects of the side effects typically disappear once the body has adjusted to the medication.

It is logical to think that preventive measures are the most effective treatment. Avoiding foods that are high in uric acid could decrease the chance of developing Gout. Limiting your consumption of alcohol is another way to reduce the risk of the development of gout.

People suffering from gout must refrain from drinking more than three drinks a day. Another way to prevent it is to cut down or eliminate purine-rich foods from your diet, such as organ meatsand sweetbreads anchovies, sardines and shrimp.

There are a variety of natural and organic products for sale. Omega 3 fatty acids as well as flax seed can reduce the damage to tissues and swelling. The burdock root can be helpful in getting rid of acid waste and for stabilizing the levels of uric acid.

If you are suffering from gout you should consult your doctor to get guidance on pain relief and the right foods to eat. Gout can be treated by a healthy diet and treatment program for pain.

Chapter 12: Treatments For Gout

Gout treatment in general usually includes one or several prescription medicines. Your physician will assess the overall health of you and your existing condition, and prescribe drugs that are most likely to give you the greatest relief. When you are suffering from attacks, you can take drugs that can be used to manage it and reduce your symptoms. Patients are often given a prescription medication to help prevent attacks in the future.

Treatments to treat attacks

There are many medications your doctor might prescribe to combat acute gout attacks, which could comprise:

A) Nonsteroidal anti-inflammatory medicines These medicines are prescribed to relieve inflammation and pain that is associated with Gout. Patients may be given an order for NSAID to treat more severe cases of inflammation. There is a chance of side effects you need to be aware of since they could be grave. They include stomach pain , and ulcers.

B) Corticosteroids: These medications help to decrease inflammation, and are stronger than nonsteroidal anti-inflammatory medicines. Doctors typically recommend corticosteroids if the patient is not able to use colchicine and NSAID drugs. There's a chance for several serious adverse consequences, such as poor healing from wounds, bone loss, which can lead to fractures of bones, and a reduction in the body's ability combat infections.

C) Colchicine: It is a painkiller and is extremely effective in relieving discomfort that is associated with gout. To get maximum relief, it is essential that you start taking this medication immediately after the onset of gout symptoms. This drug is usually recommended to people who are not able to take anti-inflammatory nonsteroidal drugs. It is normal to feel nausea, diarrhea and vomiting as well as other negative effects associated with this drug.

Medicines to treat complications

If you experience several gout attacks in the course of a year or when the attacks you experience are extremely painful, doctors may recommend treatments to decrease the risk of developing complications due to the condition. The following drugs are typically used to prevent complications from gout:

A) Xanthine oxidase inhibitors: This kind of medication works to prevent your body's production of acids. The most popular ones include the febuxostat as well as allopurinol. Gout risk and its associated complications decreases when your body produces less Uric acid. The most frequent adverse effects are the rash and nausea, but you can also suffer diminished liver function.

B) Probenecid: The medication is designed to increase the speed at which the kidneys work to eliminate uric acids from the body. This means there's less risk of uric acids accumulating and causing crystal formation. The most frequent symptoms are abdominal pain, rash and stomach however, there is also the possibility to develop kidney stones.

If gout isn't appropriately treated, complications could be experienced. Certain people may suffer from complications even though they receive correct medical treatment. The most frequent complications are kidney stones, recurrent gout and advanced Gout.

Gout Cure

While there are treatment options for gout that be effective, natural remedies for gout will help combat the symptoms, prevent further attacks, while improving your general health simultaneously. It is crucial to learn about all natural remedies because making use of them correctly is crucial. You can mix several of them since there is no chance of adverse interactions , as the case with prescription drugs. Make sure to be aware of any remedies you are trying and track the way you use these treatments.

Food and Diet

The expression 'you will be what you put into your mouth' holds relevant to your risk of developing gout. The right diet will help you treat an existing gout attack and also keep future attacks from happening. There are a variety of food items, drinks and diet changes that can assist you to get rid of gout. These are:

A) Consuming a cup of blueberries is helpful in relieving pain with Gout.

B) Cherries may help reduce pain, but they also may help lower the levels of uric acid. A small study examined women who consumed 280 grams of Bing cherries twice the course of a single day after the overnight fast. They were tested 3 hours after eating the fruit and their uric acid levels had significantly lower. Also, there was a reduction in inflammation.

C) Celery seeds aid in eliminate uric acid out of the body. Celery can also prove beneficial since it is high in amount of water and eating more fluids will help remove this acid from the body.

D) Cayenne pepper is a well-known anti-inflammatory, and due to this, it helps reduce the pain and discomfort of gout as it helps to heal. It is possible to mix it into various recipes to reap the anti-inflammatory benefit.

E) Eating a diet rich in fiber can help eliminate the body of uric acid. It is recommended to consume additional fiber from healthy sources, such as whole grains.

F) Increased levels of potassium aids in fighting gout. Include these foods in your diet every day to prevent gout and lower the chance of recurring attacks such as peaches, potatoes cantaloupe and bananas, skim milk and fat-free Yogurt the kidney bean, spinach lime beans, avocado carrots, orange juice tomatoes, and prunes.

G) Grapes can reduce your uric acids. It is possible to eat 1 cup of grapes per day to get this effect. Both red and green grapes perform in a similar way.

H) The lemon juice is able to neutralize acids like the uric acid. It does this by stimulating calcium carbonate that is present in the body. The effect is similar to those high school experiments in which baking soda was used to lower chemical acidity. Strawberries can also provide the same effect and neutralize acidity in the body.

I) It is crucial to consume a diet which is free of purines to help treat gout and avoid attacks in the future. Purines are directly linked to the development of this condition as the uric acid produced is the result of dissolving purines in the body. Reduced intake of purines will help to protect against damage caused by free radicals within your body.

J) Parsley is largely water-based and assists in flushing uric acid from the body. It helps because it has an effect of diuretic nature that encourages urine production. Because you remove uric acid through the kidneys, frequent urination results in lower levels of uric acid.

K) Quercetin is a flavonoid that treats gout by blocking the enzyme responsible for causing it. It is possible to get this flavonoid through eating apples, capers fruit, the citrus fruit, honey extracted from tea tree blossoms and onions, eucalyptus and cranberries, cherries, the leafy greens of vegetables, and raspberries.

Teas are extremely effective in helping to treat this condition. Black and green tea are popular since they are simple to locate and have flavonoid antioxidants that help to ease inflammation within the body. It is recommended to make your own tea as it ensures you're receiving the maximum benefits of antioxidants and other nutrients. Other teas that are popular for gout are:

A) Chamomile tea: This tea is great for people suffering from gout as it has three potent anti-inflammatory substances. It also reduces the risk of uric acids buildup.

B) Buchu tea: This kind of tea is used to remove uric acid crystals from the body.

C) Nettle tea Nettle tea is known for its capability to eliminate uric acids from your body. It can be consumed or apply it to your skin. If you prefer to apply it to the body you can add one to 2 teaspoons of the nettle into hot water in a cup and allow it to cool down to a temperature of lukewarm. Make a washcloth soaked in the tea made from nettle then apply the washcloth directly on the joint that is affected over a period of 30 mins.

To ensure you're receiving the maximum benefits from tea, ensure that the leaves and flowers are steeped for 5 minutes and the roots are steeped over 10 mins. This ensures that all flavonoids that fight and heal gout, are released prior to drinking the tea. Drinking between two and four cups of tea a day is suggested. You can pick only one or several of these teas every day.

Coffee could also help combat Gout. It has been proven to lower uric acids levels and this is the case for both decaffeinated and caffeinated coffee. The reason coffee causes this effect is not understood and researchers continue to research the issue. One reason regular coffee could aid is due to the fact that it contains caffeine. It is an effective diuretic that induces urination. When you pee, you're eliminating extra uric acid from the body. Since decaffeinated caffeine produces the same effects and is a little confused about the mechanism behind it currently.

All in all, you need to make a food plan that contains the essential nutrients every day. Concentrate the bulk of your food on vegetables, fruits and whole grains. It is possible to eat meat or fish, however, keep your consumption to a minimum and get your protein from other sources including soybeans and even tofu. Drink plenty of water that is filtered and be sure to drink at the minimum of up to six glasses over the course of a 24-hour period. It is vital to drink enough water as dehydration can increase the risk of Gout attacks and drinking water is essential to rid uric acids from the body.

Supplements and herbs

With regards to Gout, there are a myriad of supplements and herbs can be beneficial in getting this condition to a stop. It is important to understand what supplements are available and precisely how they could aid you. It is essential to consult your physician before adding any herbs or supplements to to ensure maximum security. This will also ensure that you are making the proper dosage and using the supplement or herb in the correct way. A proper dosage and the right administration are essential to get the best results.

Alfalfa: Alfalfa has the ability to lower the amount of uric acids in the body. This is due to it being a rich source of nutrients that support kidney function. It also has diuretic properties to remove the accumulation of fluids, like uric acids within muscles and joints. The ingredients that create this effect are carotene, phosphorus, magnesium calcium, and potassium. It also helps neutralize uric acids, fight inflammation, and supply your body with essential antioxidants. All of this works to stop uric acids from crystallizing and leading to Gout.

Vitamin B complex Vitamin B Complex supplements are extremely popular since the B vitamins are required for a variety of things within the body, for example, controlling metabolism as well as providing energy. Another important function of B vitamins is helping the body absorb Uric acid, and also make it non-toxic. This stops the acid from accumulating and causing crystals of uric acids within and around joints, ensuring that gout is not likely to develop. They are water-soluble and your kidneys are able to eliminate the ones the body doesn't require However, it is crucial to ensure that you're receiving the correct dosage.

Bilberry: Bilberry is an herb that has been extensively used to treat symptoms and treat an attack of Gout. It is able to remove gout from the body, which means people who use it will experience reduced symptoms and eliminate their gout permanently. It is also recommended to take it regularly to avoid future episodes of gout.

Black cohosh Black cohosh is often advertised as a herb that can alleviate the symptoms of menopausal however, it may also help to neutralize the acidity of blood. Additionally, because postmenopausal women are more susceptible to Gout, taking it regularly as a supplement could help in reducing the risk of gout for this population.

Bromelain: Bromelain has powerful anti-inflammatory properties, which means it can combat swelling, stiffness and pain that are associated with Gout. It is also able to help treat gout by reducing inflammation that occurs in the body. It is essential not to combine this herb with blood thinner drugs.

Devil's claw: This plant is great for relieving discomfort and inflammation associated with Gout. It also helps lower the amount of uric acids in the body. It is not recommended to mix this herb with blood thinners.

Cat's claw: Cat's cube has many health benefits and can aid in reducing gout symptoms, such as improving your immune system and decreasing inflammation, and possessing antifungal as well as antibacterial properties. This herb could cause an increase in the leukemia or autoimmune disorder and those suffering from such conditions should avoid this herb and opt for an alternative to treat their gout, to ensure security and efficacy.

Turmeric: Turmeric is well-known for its potent properties in combating inflammation. It can help in curing an attack of gout and decrease the severity of symptoms as it resolves. The herb has the effect of reducing blood flow, therefore it is crucial to avoid using it in conjunction with blood thinners.

DMSO: DMSO, or dimethylsulfoxide is a chemical that plays a crucial function in reducing inflammation within the body. It can also help dissolve the uric acid crystals and help treat gout-related symptoms.

Oils from fish: These oils have essential fatty acids which are vital to overall well-being. They play a significant function in reducing inflammation within the body. This may help with gout since Gout can cause extreme amounts of inflammation.

Folic acid Folic acid is a vital B vitamin that aids in regulate metabolism and energy levels. For gout, this vitamin can be helpful in reducing levels of uric acid within the body. A lower level of uric acids reduces the chance of joints becoming gouty.

Hawthorn: Hawthorn helps to accelerate the speed at which someone recovers from an attack of gout. It is recommended to take it when you first notice gout in order to heal it quicker and in reducing the symptoms.

Hydrangea: Many people have heard of Hydrangea as a flower however, it can be consumed as a natural supplement. In the case of gout, it helps to lower inflammation levels, which helps reduce pain and treat attacks of gout.

L-glutamine: It is the most abundant amino acid, and the body produces sufficient quantities. However, in conditions of stress or extreme stress, like in the case of a gout attack the body might require greater amounts of the amino acid that it can make by itself. This supplement is a natural antiacid which makes it useful in neutralizing acids such as the uric acid in the body.

L-glutathione: The body naturally produces these substances and people can get more of it from their diets when they consume fruits and vegetables. It is a supplement that can be taken to boost the speed and effectively the body can eliminate uric acid from the body.

L-glycine acids is one that your body could use other chemicals to produce. L-glycine can neutralize acids through its anti-acid effects.

L-methionine: This amino acids is vital for a wide range of cell functions inside the body. This supplement aids in detoxifying purines and prevent the rise of levels of uric acids in the body.

Nettle: If you would prefer to avoid nettle tea or in topical form it is possible to take the supplement in herbal form. As a supplement it can still reduce the amount of uric acid within your body , preventing crystallization and accumulation.

Red clover: The red clover does not directly target gout like many other supplements and herbs. It instead plays the general function of removing toxic substances from the body. This assists in the elimination of excess uric acids so that it's not able to build up within the body and cause crystallization.

Saffron: Saffron is a exquisite spice that you can use in a variety recipes to impart an unique taste. Incorporating saffron into your food at least a couple of times each week can aid in the treatment and stop the development of gout. This spice is advantageous as it helps to regulate level of the uric acids within the body.

Shark cartilage Shark cartilage is believed to be very beneficial to joints. This applies to a joint which is affected by Gout. It helps to improve the general health of the joint, and also reduce any pain that is associated with it.

Spearmint: Spearmint is a natural and effective soother that is used internally and topically for Gout. To use it internally you can prepare your own tea or consume a supplement made of spearmint. If you are looking to use this herb on your skin it is necessary to create compresses. Make a tea of fresh spearmint leaves, and then simmer them with boiling water 5 minutes, then remove from the heat. When the mixture reaches an lukewarm temperature, you can put a washcloth into it, and apply it onto the joint that is affected for approximately 30 minutes. If you decide to apply the herb internally, externally or both, spearmint can ease Gout pain.

Vitamin C Vitamin C: This vitamin helps to reduce the amount of uric acids within the body. Adults should consume around 90 mg of vitamin C each day, while women of adult age are supposed to get 75 milligrams of this vitamin every daily. This helps to avoid deficiency and ensure that the uric acid levels in the body remain within control. If someone is looking to boost their vitamin C levels above the recommended daily levels it is recommended to consult an expert first to ensure that it is done in a safe manner.

Vitamin E: People who suffer from an vitamin E deficiency are at greater risk of developing Gout. This is because of an insufficient supply that causes the formation of crystals of uric acids. Adults should consume 15 milligrams each throughout the day. You can get supplements or include more vitamin E into your diet. The best sources of this vitamin are the wheat germ oil and almonds sunflower seeds, peanut butter and Safflower oil.

Don't take in more daily doses in vitamin A and Niacin. Both are believed to cause Gout attack. Eat a varied diet to absorb these vitamins and don't consume any supplements that have these nutrients.

When choosing the herbal supplements and herbs to treat gout that you're planning to take there are a few aspects to be aware of. Be sure you're using a brand that is reputable and has a an established reputation for producing high-quality products. Review the research findings to determine if the product or ingredient is suitable for your needs. Look over the label of the bottle attentively and follow the dosage guidelines exactly unless your physician has given you specific dosage and dosage instructions.

Because different people respond differently to different doses of medication It is advised to talk with a doctor or a seasoned herbalist for a dosage that's right for you for your gout, as well as your general health.

A few people also get relief from gout using different remedies made from homeopathy. Gout homeopathy can be used as an aid to treat the symptoms , while the supplements, herbs, and other treatments are relieving the condition. If you're taking homeopathy, the typical dosage is between three and five 30C to 12X pellets. The recommended dosage is every 1 to 4 hours, according to the dosage instructions given by the homeopath. Homeopathic remedies to treat symptoms of gout are:

A) Aconite treatment is recommended for painful and swelling joints as well as suddenly burning pain.

B) Berberis vulgaris: This remedy can help lessen the pain that gout can cause when walking.

C) Colchicum: This may help to ease the discomfort caused by gout that is associated with change in weather.

D) Rhus toxicodendron: This homeopathic remedy is prescribed for joints which are hot and swollen and stiff and painful.

(e.g.) Belladonna: This remedy is used to treat throbbing pain as well as hot joint.

F) Bryonia could help with pain related to motion.

G) The Ledum method is typically employed when a joint affected by gout is purple or is swollen.

Home Remedies

There are numerous home remedies with gout. These remedies help treat it by changing the body's structure in a manner that does not favor the buildup of uric acid. If uric acid isn't built up, crystals will not form , and gout is not a possibility. Each of the solutions at home can be combined to get the best results.

Apple cider vinegar The apple cider vinegar is a great option to use externally and internally to fight Gout. If you are taking apples cider vinegar in the body the uric acid crystal pH gets altered, and the body is able to eliminate them. It is also possible to soak your joint in the affected area to ease pain and inflammation. If you're drinking apples cider vinegar for internal use, you should take one tablespoon and place it into 8 glasses of water for drinking. Do this 3 times per every day.

Baking soda Baking soda can be described as an alkali. when you acidize it to an acidic substance it reduces its acidity. This is the process that baking soda performs to the uric acids in the body. It also helps in alkalizing the whole body. Because baking soda has an extremely strong flavor It is recommended to add 1 teaspoon to non-acidic juice. Take care of the amount you are taking in as excessive alkalizing the body can cause harm.

Iceapplication directly to the joint affected is one of the most simple home remedies , and it can work. Ice is a great way to reduce the pain and inflammation that is associated with Gout. If you apply ice, you must ensure that you don't apply it directly on your skin. A washcloth should be placed in between you and your skin in order to avoid burning from ice. Let the ice remain in position for about 15 to 20 minutes before removing it. If you're applying frequent ice, be sure to allow for 30 minutes between each application. Ideally, you should apply ice three or four every day to help reduce swelling and pain related to gout.

Rest The joint that is affected is essential because if persist in using it in the course of the course of a gout attack this can delay the attack and worsen the discomfort. When the pain has lessened and you are able to rest, you must take a break and rest your joint, elevating it with a pillow. Avoid placing pressure on the joint for as long as you can and ensure it stays up all day. If you are going to bed in the evening, be aware of your sleeping habits and be sure not to allow sheets or blankets to press on the joint that is affected. It is usually recommended to keep the joint free of blankets and sheets.

Lifestyle Changes

Your lifestyle can have a significant influence upon your health overall as well as your risk of developing gout. It is possible to treat your gout problem by making the necessary adjustments to your life. The following lifestyle modifications are usually advised to all sufferers. The most frequent lifestyle changes that can help in curing gout attacks and prevent future attacks are:

A) Eliminate drinking alcohol entirely, especially when you are suffering from an acute Gout attack. Drinking less alcohol can lessen the amount of purines that your body requires to breakdown.

b) limit the amount of you eat of fish, poultry, or meat you consume. In general, you shouldn't consume more than 4 to 6 inches of food each day. The foods listed above contain moderate levels of purines. This is a substance you must reduce if you have Gout.

C) Drink between two and four daily liters of fluid. The majority of this is plain water. This assists in flushing the excess uric acids out of your body.

D) Be aware of your intake of protein and ensure it's at a moderate level throughout the day. It is recommended to make the most portion of the protein you consume from food sources which are nutritious, such as tofu, nuts eggs, dairy products, and eggs that are free of fat or low in calories.

e) Discuss with your doctor about implementing the process of losing weight when you're overweight. people who have excess body weight are more likely to have greater levels of uric acids. Therefore, if you are able to shed weight, you could as well reduce the amount of uric acids in your body.

f) It is important to be active on a regular basis that is, working out every day of the week for minimum 30 minutes at a time. This can aid in preventing Gout, as well as reduce your weight, one of the factor that can increase your gout risk.

Because your liver and kidneys also play an important role in determining whether or not you develop gout, it is important to adopt all necessary lifestyle adjustments to ensure that both the organs are in good health. The lifestyle modifications that help promote healthy kidneys as well as a healthy liver include:

A) Intensifying your daily intake of water

B) Consuming foods that assist in preventing gout attacks and treat the current attack

c) Eliminating any excess weight

d) Eliminating alcohol such as beer and other types that contain alcohol out of your daily diet

E) Limiting all food items which can raise the level of uric acids within the body

Chapter 13: Healthy Breakfasts For Gout...

1 - Steel Cut Oats

This isn't your grandmother's oatmeal, nor is it an easy breakfast made with instant oatmeal. The steel cut oats contain intact oat germ as well as cut kernels. They're digested less quickly than other oatmeal varieties and therefore you'll have more nutrients from them.

Serves 3-4 people.

Prep and cooking time 45 minutes

Ingredients:

Three cups of drinking water filtering

1. Cup of oatmeal * 1 cup of oats, steel cut

* 1/4 cup blueberries frozen

Half banana ripe , but not too ripe

1. 1/4 cup of walnuts crushed

* Milk, skim

* Butter Organic

* Syrup, maple syrup

* Cinnamon * Ground

* Salt sea

Instructions:

1. Bring three cups of water to a boiling. Include 1 cup steel-cut oats and one pinch of sea salt.

2. Once the water is back to the point of boiling, reduce the heat and let it simmer for half an hour. Cover the pot with a lid and stir it occasionally.

3. Once you're close to finishing Add the walnuts, 1 tablespoon butter, chopped blueberries and bananas. Mix until everything is well and hot.

4. Put a few scoops of oatmeal into a bowl and add milk to give the oatmeal a creamy texture. Add 1 pinch of ground cinnamon, and a little maple syrup. Serve.

2. Berry Cherry Smoothie

Cherries have a lower chance of gout attacks than other fruits that you could mix into smoothies. The low-fat or non-fat dairy products are less purine than dairy products that are full-fat also. Therefore, cherries with skim milk and low fat yogurt can make an ideal gout-friendly breakfast smoothie.

Serves 2 people

Prep and cooking time 10 minutes

Ingredients:

1 cup cherries with tart, pitted and frozen

Half cup of milk skim

1 cup yogurt plain, low-fat

* 2 tbsp. of blueberries, freshly

* 1 tbsp. in concentrated cherries juice

* 1 tbsp. of honey organic

* 1/2 tsp. of vanilla extract, pure

8.8 Cubes Ice

Instructions:

1. In a food processor, add the ingredients and blend until the mixture is smooth. 2. Pour smoothie into 2 glasses. Add the cherries. Serve.

3 - Pumpkin Walnut Pancakes

Cayenne aids in reducing elimination, while bananas aid the body to become alkaline. Protein is derived through nut butters and nuts. Overall this is a healthy meal that will fill you up as well.

Serves up to 1-2 servings

Prep + Cooking Time 50 minutes

Ingredients:

* 1/2 cup pumpkin, canned

1 cup yogurt plain

Half cup of nuts chopped

* 1 banana that is perfectly ripe

* 1/4 tsp. of baking soda, no aluminum

* 1 yolk of an egg taken from a large egg

* 14 cup of the flour whole wheat

4. Egg whites made from large eggs

* 1/4 tsp. of salt sea

* 1/4 tsp. cayenne

* Butter organic

Pure maple syrup.

Instructions:

1. In a large bowl, whisk in pumpkin, yogurt flour, egg yolk and baking soda.

2. Separately, mix egg whites with sea salt, cayenne and cayenne together. Blend this into the yogurt mixture.

3. Large skillet should be heated to medium. heat. In a skillet, melt some butter. Scoop 1/3 cup of the batter into your skillet per pancake. When they're cooked and crisp flip them over to fry the on the other side.

4. After pancakes have been cooked then spread butter over them. Lay banana slices on top. Add a small amount of maple syrup. Serve. Gout-friendly recipes for lunches and Dinners, as well as Side Dishes and appetizers

4 - Onion-Herb-Soup

It's a very simple soup recipe and it's a fantastic comfort food that can help you get rid of your sinuses and calm your stomach. You'll be able to enjoy it when you're in good health, too.

Serves 3-5 people

Prep and Cooking Time: 1 and 1/2 hours

Ingredients:

* 3 onions sliced Large

* 4 shallots cut into slices

* 4 tbsp. of olive oil and olive

* 1 tbsp. of rosemary dried

* 1 tsp. of thyme dried

Two cups of water water that has been filtered

Four cups vegetable broth, with low sodium

* One pinch black pepper ground black

4. 6 to 8 pieces of bread white

4. 4 pieces of cheese low-fat thin

Instructions:

1. In a soup pot, heat oil. Once it is hot add shallot and onions. Stir. Cook them for 15 to 20 minutes. Onions will begin to caramelize.

2. Add the ground rosemary, pepper, and thyme. Add vegetable stock as well as water.

3. Let soup cook for about an hour on medium. heat.

4. Pour the soup of onions into separate bowls. Decorate them with slices bread and cheese slices.

5. Set bowls in the oven. Bake for 5-10 minutes or until cheese is melt.

6. Serve warm.

5. 5 - The New Waldorf Salad

The latest Waldorf salad makes use of low-fat mayonnaise, accompanied by nuts, celery dried cranberries, apples, and much more. It's a bit like the original recipe and helps in reducing appetite during the afternoon.

Serves 4.

Prep and cooking time 15 minutes

Ingredients:

* 2 tbsp. of mayonnaise, low-fat

* 1 tbsp. from lemon juice freshly squeezed If there is any

Two cubed apple slices small

1. Cup of seedless, halved grapes Red

13 cup of dried cranberries dried

1. 1/4 cup walnuts chopped finely

1. 1 celery stalk cut thinly

8. Leaves of Bibb (or Boston lettuce

Instructions:

1. Mix the lemon juice and mayonnaise in a medium-sized bowl.

2. Add apples, cranberries and grapes to mix.

3. Add the walnuts and celery. Mix thoroughly. 4. Serve on beds consisting of 2 lettuce leaves per person. Serve.

6 - Zucchini Cheese Casserole

Your family and you will enjoy this easy casserole! It's delicious and has the flavor of cheese, and is also low in carbs. It's a wonderful food item to serve as a side dish. Even kids love it!

Four servings are served.

Prep + Cooking Time: 1 hour and 40 minutes

* 2 lbs. of zucchini

*1 chopped onion large

* 1/3 cup rice long-grain, uncooked

*1 can soup made from cream of mushrooms Low-fat

* 2 eggs, beaten

* 2 tbsp. of butter, unalted

* 1 cup cheddar cheese, reduced fat grated

Instructions:

1. Preheat the oven to 350F.

2. Cut zucchini and onion into pieces.

3. Sauté the zucchini and onion in a light sauté.

4. While they sauté in the pan, add eggs as well as soup, butter, and rice into a large bowl.

5. Add onion and zucchini to the rice mix.

6. Mix thoroughly. Pour into medium sized casserole dish. Sprinkle with cheese.

7. Bake at 350F for about an hour. Serve.

7 - - Cabbage Pasta

Cabbage and pasta work well for a side dish or even as a light meal all on its own. I've removed the bacon from in the recipe in order to ensure it is gout-friendly. If you love vegetables, you'll appreciate how simple this dish is for a weekday evening after work.

Cooks for 4-6 servings

Prep + Cooking Time 1 hour plus 2-3 hours of chilling time

* 3 Cups of Pasta gemelli

Three cups red cabbage shred

* 2 carrots shredded medium

* 1 and 1/2 cups salad dressing, garlic roasted with a smooth

Instructions:

1. Boil water in a large pan. Cook pasta according to the instructions on the package and then drain it.

2. Mix the remaining ingredients in a large bowl. Add cooked pasta. Stir gently.

3. Cool for 2 to 3 hours before serving.

8 Balsamic Chicken

This balsamic-based glaze adds flavor to the chicken dish. Balsamic vinegar is much more beneficial than regular vinegar. The chicken is succulent and tender and delicious.

Four servings are served.

Prep and cooking time 40 minutes + 2 - 4 hours of time to marinate

4. Chicken breasts Boneless

* 1/2 cup oil, olive

* 1/2 cup vinegar, balsamic

• 1 to 2 cloves of garlic Crushed

Instructions:

1. Combine vinegar, garlic, and oil in a large container with a zippered top.

2. Add chicken. Seal the bag and place in fridge for two to four hours.

3. Grill or bake chicken until fully cooked. Serve.

9 - Parmesan Cheesy Noodles

A lot of pasta recipes sound delicious, however they can be difficult to prepare. After a long day at work or in a hurry it's not always easy to find the time to cook dishes such as that. Although this recipe is easy, it's quite satisfying.

Serves 4.

* 1 lb. of noodles, fine

*1 cup Parmesan cheese reduced in fat grated

* 2 cloves of crushed garlic

* 4 tbsp. of fresh coriander chopped

* 6 tbsp. of olive oil and olive

* 3/4 tsp. of salt, salt that is kosher.

* 1/2 tsp. of black pepper ground

Instructions:

1. Prepare the noodles following the directions on the package.

2. As the noodles cook chop the coriander. In a large bowl, add coriander.

3. After cooking is done take noodles off and pour into bowls with coriander.

4. Mix all the ingredients in a well-coordinated manner. Blend them into noodles. Serve warm.

10, Pear with Spinach Salad

It will take you about 30 minutes to throw the delicious salad. The dressing is classic tart and is a great dish to serve with a dinner.

Serves up to 4-6 servings

*4 cups of leaves from spinach baby

2 sliced pears, mature

1 1/2 lemons, freshly juice only

* 1 tbsp. of olive oil and olive

* 1 tbsp. of mustard, Dijon

* One pinch of black pepper ground

Instructions:

1. Place spinach leaves on a platter. Serve them on top with slices of pears.

2. Mix oil, ground pepper lemon juice, mustard and oil in a small Jar. Close the lid, and shake vigorously.

3. Pour dressing over salad. Blend gently. Serve.

Conclusion

Gout does not appear to be a common illness. It can affect everyone. It can strike even while you sleep. It is also possible in the case of young. There are numerous studies done to treat gout and there are individuals who are able to maintain their well-being. They bounced back from an attack, and take control of their lives once more.

It's better said than done, I'm sure. But, it's up to you to make your decision. This book is only an instruction manual to help you deal with your illness. All the work will be handled by you. It is my opinion that the foremost thing you need to keep in mind in this case is that the fact that gout can be avoided. The most important thing to do is take the initial steps to prevent. Check with your physician and live an, healthy and active life.

www.ingramcontent.com/pod-product-compliance
Lightning Source LLC
Chambersburg PA
CBHW071654030426
R18080400001B/R180804PG42336CBX00002B/3